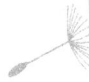

I0091079

PRAISE FOR *LOVE'S LAST ACT*

"It is 'Love's Last Act' indeed to leave those you love free of regrets [concerning your medical care in your final months and years]. This wise, beautiful, deceptively simple book will give you all the information you need—and not too much!—to navigate your later years successfully and prepare for a well-supported death on your own terms. This handbook is deeply informed by Deborah Price's years of clinical practice, education, wisdom, and dare I say, love. Highly recommended."

—Katy Butler, Author,
Knocking on Heaven's Door
and *The Art of Dying Well*

"This book so aptly reflects the author's deep skill, wisdom and compassionate caring offered over decades to so many at the end of their lives. Her profound respect and love for life has inspired her to give readers a clear, honest and thorough roadmap for navigating a topic that can often be frightening and confusing. I couldn't agree more with Ms. Price that planning for one's care at the end of life well ahead of when it is needed is a profound and lasting gift to your loved ones. And *Love's Last Act* is indeed a gift to all who peruse its pages."

—Carole O'Toole,
Integrative Oncology Navigator and
Author, *Healing Outside the Margins: The Survivor's Guide to Integrative Cancer Care*

LOVE'S
LAST ACT

PLANNING A
PEACEFUL DEATH
WITH NO REGRETS

DEBORAH PRICE, RN, MSN

This publication contains the opinions and ideas of its author. It is intended to provide helpful and informative material on the subjects addressed in the publication. It is sold with the understanding that the author and publisher are not rendering medical, health, or any other kind of personal professional services in the book. The reader should consult his or her medical, health, or other competent professional before adopting any of the suggestions in this book or drawing inferences from it.

The author and publisher specifically disclaim all responsibility for any liability, loss, or risk, personal or otherwise that is incurred as a consequence, directly or indirectly, of the use and application of any of the contents of this book.

Some names and identifying characteristics have been changed.

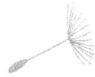

To Every Body
May you live your life to the fullest
and may your death be one of comfort and peace.

TABLE OF CONTENTS

A STORY TO CONSIDER

B ill, age 72, took a fall off a ladder while cleaning leaves out of his roof gutters. He was transported to the hospital via ambulance for a suspected broken hip. Bill was somewhat overweight, with high blood pressure, and in the early stages of Parkinson's disease. Because of the tremors in his hands, Bill was proud to say he had recently quit smoking. All in all, Bill considered himself a regular guy in average health.

The X-ray done in the emergency room confirmed that his right hip was fractured. Bill would be admitted and surgery scheduled. As standard practice, the ER nurse asked Bill if he had signed a "living will" or if he wanted a Do Not Resuscitate (DNR) order should his heart or breathing stop during his hospitalization. Bill did not have a living will. He accepted the pamphlet that explained the DNR order, but did not sign the form. Bill's wife, Betty, also read the information and accepted her husband's decision not to sign the form at that time.

The hip surgery was successful. The orthopedic surgeon suggested a neurological consult to adjust the medication for Bill's Parkinson's disease. Bill's adjustment to new meds was complicated by a post-op fever that sapped his strength. The physical therapy required for his hip was repeatedly delayed as Bill remained in bed. He received frequent respiratory treatments but developed pneumonia that seemed to defy therapy. He grew progressively weaker, yet neither Bill, his wife, nor the medical team ever discussed again what Bill would want should his heart or breathing stop.

A random accident, falling off a ladder, and now Bill languished in a hospital bed, his strength dwindling. One morning at 5 a.m. during her routine hourly check, the night nurse, Donna, discovered Bill not breathing and had no pulse. She immediately pressed the button on his bed to alert the Code Blue resuscitation team, loudly shouted for help, and began cardiopulmonary resuscitation (CPR). Another floor nurse joined her and took over administering oxygen. In less than two minutes, Bill's room was teeming with staff as the Code Blue team arrived with their large Code Cart equipped with life-saving drugs and a defibrillator.

The Code team quickly took command, rolling Bill to one side to place a backboard beneath him, then stripped him of his gown before commencing chest compressions. Lying naked on the bed, Bill was surrounded by the

Code Blue team. A tube was placed in Bill's trachea to help open his airway and reestablish regular breathing. A critical care nurse applied EKG leads that confirmed his heart could be shocked back into an effective rhythm and the Code team leader applied the defibrillator paddles. The first two attempts failed but the third shock restored Bill's heartbeat. Medications were injected through his intravenous line. The Code Blue team was able to stabilize him, but there was no way of knowing exactly how long Bill had been without a heartbeat or breathing, and Bill remained unconscious.

Transferred to intensive care, with heartbeat and breathing stabilized mechanically, Bill stayed unresponsive. For days, Betty sat at his bedside hoping he would open his eyes, but Bill remained in a coma. After many tests and repeated clinical and imaging studies, the neurologist determined that Bill was in a permanent vegetative state.

Heartbroken and bereft, Betty finally agreed to have Bill transferred to a long-term care facility equipped to care for him. Unfortunately, the facility was far from their home. Frail and alone, Betty was left to determine by herself what her husband would have wanted in these circumstances. Would he have wanted her to remain his caregiver in his present state or would he have accepted suspension of life-sustaining measures?

Betty could not believe this was happening.

Could this scenario happen to you?

If you were Bill or Betty, would you have made different decisions? If so, when?

PREFACE

This guide is intended for every body who is going to die, regardless of how and when death occurs. Of course, we know that every one of us will die. When and if we ever do think about our eventual death, we envision the peaceful death often depicted in movies and television shows. Yet the sad truth is that very few of us actually experience a death of comfort and peace. Why? Because we do not actively plan for our inevitable death. Even when diagnosed with a life-limiting illness, we are much more likely to choose aggressive treatments instead of considering comfort care measures.

The good news is that today death can be more comfortable and peaceful, than many people realize, not only for the person who is dying but for all those left behind. When family and friends witness the peace and comfort experienced by their dying loved one, it can ease their grief and sorrow. Life is hard enough to face going forward in their loved one's absence, but it is so much harder to bear the loss if final memories are ones of wretched pain or if there are regrets about how the final illness was handled.

After nearly half a century of being a nurse in acute care settings, in oncology and clinical research trials, elder care and assisted living, and hospice, my heart and my head compel me to write about the act and the art of dying. It is my sincere hope that this book will help my fellow humans truly consider how they want to live to their dying day and how they can care for loved ones through a final illness. To me, the ultimate last act of love for yourself and those you love is to fully consider and actively plan for the death experience you hope to have. It is my fervent prayer that by doing this essential planning, you and those you love will experience a peaceful death, unburdened by needless, painful regrets.

LOVE'S
LAST ACT

Youth is a gift of Nature, but Age is a work of Art.
Stanislaw Jercy Lec

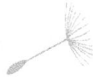

CHAPTER 1

HOW TO THRIVE AS YOU AGE

B efore we talk about dying, let's talk about living—
and living well. I think we all can agree that while
we are here on Earth, we want to enjoy life. One way to
do so is to accept that we are aging.

Aging is a normal, natural lifelong process. When
we are young, we call it "growth and development." We
celebrate each milestone as babies grow into toddlers,
toddlers to teens, teens to twenty-something adults. We
seem to stop celebrating after that though, and don't look
at aging as the gift it is. As the saying goes, do not regret
growing older; it is a privilege denied to many.

Most of us when we are young are vibrant and
healthy. Visits to the doctor are perfunctory with annual
physical exams and when we get sick, we go to the
doctor—or these days, a nurse practitioner (NP) or physician assistant (PA)—who may provide a prescription

or instructions for how we can return to good general health. Medical care is fairly easy and life goes on. As we continue to age, that brings changes. Normal changes.

According to the Centers for Disease Control (CDC), age-related biologic functions peak by the age of 30 and then begin to decline. This is not "bad" news, just a fact. The slow decline in function has little impact on our daily lives. You might not notice much change except for not being able to stay up all night and party like when you were in your twenties. And now that we are a little bit older, we don't want to do that anyway!

We all know that heredity, environment, and individual experiences greatly impact our bodies and minds as we grow from infancy into adulthood and all throughout our lives, however, certain physical and mental changes occur purely from the natural aging process. For all of us. It is normal for hair to thin and turn grey. Our skin wrinkles and sags. If we do not remain active, our bodies lose muscle mass and strength, bones become more fragile, and joints become stiffer. If we do not exercise and eat a healthy diet, our arteries may stiffen so our hearts have to work harder to pump oxygen through our bodies. Our appetites and weight change as digestion slows and taste buds shrink. Our bladders become less elastic so urine may leak when we laugh, cough, or sneeze. (You're not alone if this has happened to you!)

The list goes on. Our vision becomes less acute; reading fine print becomes more difficult. Cataracts may develop, diminishing our sight in bright sunshine and causing the halo glare of lights while driving at night. Hearing may diminish so conversing with others in a crowded room becomes strenuous and tiring. "What did you say?" is a question we begin to repeat more often to our family and friends. Our sleep patterns change. We may wake once or twice (or more) during the night, often because we need to use the bathroom. If we do not work to remain active, we may notice more difficulty maintaining balance when walking, getting into the tub, or climbing stairs. We may also experience more difficulty juggling multiple tasks that we did with ease when we were younger. We might have difficulty remembering the name of someone we just met, why we walked into a room in search of something, or where we left our reading glasses. All of this is normal.

Any of that sound familiar? Nothing is wrong with you. You are simply aging! Like everyone else on the planet, our bodies change. There is no point in denying that we are aging. And as we age, we can learn to THRIVE.

Take, for example, Sam who looks in the mirror while brushing his teeth and bemoans his receding hairline and belly paunch. He turns on the TV and plops onto the couch with a bowl of pretzels. Then he goes and grabs a beer. Sally eyes herself in the mirror and smiles at her gray hair as she puts on lipstick before heading out to meet friends at exercise class. Who would you rather be like?

There are different ways to describe aging.

- Chronologic age is simply your age in years. Though there is no specific age when we become old or elderly, chronologic age helps predict the likelihood of emerging health problems.

- Biologic age is your age based on your body's response to your individual lifestyle, habits, and health history. Being active, handling stress in healthy ways, eating sensibly, limiting alcohol intake, and not smoking tobacco or using recreational drugs are habits that help your body stay more youthful. Conversely, a sedentary lifestyle, overindulging in food, liquor, and being burdened by stress makes us age faster than our chronological years. Lifestyle choices make some people biologically old well before turning 65 while others remain biologically young in their 70's and 80's. (Think about Sam and Sally above.)

- Psychologic or Functional age is how you feel physically, emotionally and socially. Those of any age who battle multiple chronic conditions or have low physical energy or emotional stamina may be considered psychologically old. People who are able to be socially active, continue working or participate in multiple arenas despite their age in years are more likely to be psychologically or functionally young.

Pete mentors a young boy, Jack, who has hereditary "brittle bone" disease. Jack has had numerous surgeries during his childhood and is primarily wheelchair bound. Though he is only nine years old chronologically, Jack's functional age exceeds that of Pete, his 63-year-old mentor.

You probably can think of many examples of people who seem "young" for their age, (Jane Fonda, for one), and the opposite, someone who is chronologically young but acts old. Sally is 65 in chronological age, but her biological age and functional age are much younger. I have always been fascinated by the aging that occurs in our nation's presidents during their terms in office. The incredible stress that this office incurs is remarkably evident in the photographs taken between the inauguration and the end of the president's term. So age may be relative, (and you can say you are as young as you feel), but aging is a fact of life.

Perhaps we see aging differently now because overall average life expectancy has greatly increased in the past century. The generation of Americans who grew up during the Great Depression and fought in WWII became of age in their teens, seen as adults by the time they graduated from high school, were "over the hill" when they turned forty, and deemed officially old at age 65, the year of retirement established by the Social Security Administration in 1935. At that time, not many people lived to be 65. The majority of the Baby Boomer generation born between 1946 and 1964 reached adulthood in their early to mid-twenties, with their careers and families established later in life than their parents' generation. Today many "Boomers" continue to work well beyond age 65. We are the generation who have strived to remain forever young.

"Young" is what you make of it. Today's life expectancy is most influenced by lifestyle habits, heredity, and healthcare. The genes you inherit from your family can increase or decrease the risk of developing a disorder that affects your longevity, but never forget that your lifestyle greatly impacts your life expectancy. Boosting your physical and emotional health through diet, exercise, and social contacts and avoiding environmental toxins, tobacco, excess alcohol or drugs helps maximize your functionality and helps prevent the development of disease. Healthcare is also a key factor. Access to good health care for wellness checks to prevent illness and also to quickly treat acute infections or potentially chronic illness helps to prolong your life. As we contemplate prolonging life, what we really are talking about is living well while we are alive. We want to FEEL GOOD as we age. And we can.

Research suggests that many health issues we encounter as we age are actually not due to the normal aging process, but are the result of our lifestyle—behavior, diet, and environment. That is very good news, since we can modify each of those elements to help maintain our good health. The decision is up to you.

To remain healthy, you can choose to:

- Make regular physical activity a fun priority by choosing something that you enjoy
  - weight-bearing exercise to build bones and keep muscles supple such as lifting free weights or the machines at the health club
  - aerobic exercise such as running, walking, jogging, cycling, swimming, or dance fitness such as Zumba
  - stretching and flexibility through Yoga or Pilates
- Reduce stress through meditation, massage, music/art therapy, hobbies
- Eat well without overindulging; increase fluids to help avoid constipation
- Limit alcohol consumption
- Not smoke or use tobacco or vaping products; avoid second-hand smoke
- Get adequate sleep

Aging with Chronic Illness

That said, normal aging often brings with it chronic health conditions and thus managing your health becomes a little more complicated. To combat the effects of these chronic conditions, doctors often prescribe medications. Then something else develops and you are back to the doctor again. As chronic conditions mount, we tend to be seen by more than one doctor who each prescribe more medicine to control our symptoms and help us remain active. With each additional medication, the risk of drug interactions increases and doctor visits might too. And the cycle goes on.

Chronic diseases are the leading cause of death in the U.S. today. Chronic illness is defined as any condition that lasts for a year or more, affects your ability to do the normal things of everyday life (dressing, eating, housekeeping), and requires frequent visits to your doctor. These include cardiovascular disease (heart disease); cancer; chronic lung disease such as emphysema, chronic obstructive pulmonary disease (COPD), aspiration pneumonia; stroke including brain bleeds or blockage; diabetes including insulin-dependent (Type I) or controlled by diet or oral hypoglycemic medications (Type II); chronic kidney disease; and dementia including Alzheimer's disease and multi-infarct dementia.

The normal changes in our bodies as we age make us more susceptible to developing chronic illness. For instance, when we're older, blood sugar levels increase more after eating carbohydrates. While the temporary increase is considered normal, if blood sugar exceeds a certain level, diabetes is diagnosed. Mild decline in mental function as we age is normal. We are often irritated by our decreased attention span, increased forgetfulness, or difficulty learning something new, but all of those things are a normal part of aging. True dementia is marked by more severe memory loss such as completely forgetting entire events, difficulty doing everyday tasks, or not recognizing loved ones or familiar surroundings.

The National Council on Aging (NCOA) estimates that approximately 80% of older adults live with at least one chronic physical illness and nearly as many cope with at least two. In 2013, the NCOA recognized that although we are taught from childhood how to be successful as adults, most of us do not know how to age well. In fact, they have created programs all about aging that I find helpful and recommend to everyone. Please get more information and learn about the NCOA's Aging Mastery Program® (AMP) at https://www.ncoa.org/healthy-aging/aging-mastery-program/.

What about you? Do you think you know how to age well? According to AARP, the Baby Boomer generation who began turning 65 in 2011 is likely the most technically savvy, forward-thinking generation of adults—who actively dismiss aging. Boomers do not like to be labeled as old and therefore "dismissible." This age group hates ageism (fear of being dismissed due to age). Boomers expect today's medical advances and technology to help them live longer and they tend to seek more medical attention for their symptoms. Their search for the fountain of youth continues, but is that realistic? Healthy? Does being in denial feel peaceful? Not to me.

Slow Medicine

In her book, *The Art of Dying Well: A Practical Guide to a Good End of Life*, award-winning science journalist Katy Butler provides several common-sense checklists to help us navigate the physical, emotional, spiritual, and financial changes that aging brings. There is a natural "slowing down" process through the years of adulthood. Butler advises that as we slow down, we reconsider our health patterns and our healthcare care team.

Rather than continuing in the realm of "fast medicine" (i.e., the tests, the drugs, the treatments, the elective surgeries, the eternal quest to remain youthful), she recommends adopting "slow medicine." Slow medicine is a philosophy from Italian physician Alberta Dolaro and popularized in the U.S. in 2008 by Dr. Dennis McCullough, a geriatrician at Dartmouth Medical School. Dr. McCullough's slow medicine emphasizes minimal medical intervention and protection from over-treatment.

One aspect of slow medicine is reviewing and reducing the number of prescriptions and over-the-counter (OTC) drugs we take. Today, it is common to see and hear many commercials for prescription drugs, OTC medications, and dietary supplements.

We are constantly told to "talk with our doctor" about adding a new medicine to the arsenal of products described to help us live happier, healthier lives. However, more medication does not guarantee better health as we age. (And how about the long list of side effects on all those commercials?!)

The plain and simple truth is that the more drugs we take, the more we risk serious drug interactions or errors in drug dosages. A study of polypharmacy (multiple medication use) in older adults published in 2015 by the Journal of Gerontology reported that between 1988 and 2010 the median number of prescription medications used among adults aged 65 and older doubled, and the proportion of older adults taking five or more medications tripled. Researchers have found that higher medication use was also associated with greater functional limitations, more falls, and greater degree of confusion or memory problems. Having multiple doctors increases our risk of taking multiple drugs. In aging, the theory of "more is better" definitely does not apply.

So how do we avoid the risks of taking multiple medications? Set up an appointment with your primary doctor, a geriatrician, or a pharmacist knowledgeable about older adults to review all medications and dietary supplements to make sure every drug or supplement you take is absolutely necessary. The aim is to make sure you and your doctor know:

- the purpose of each drug or supplement you are taking
- the dose and time you take each drug

- potential side effects
- potential drug interactions

Such a review may very well simplify your drug regimen. As research has shown, the fewer drugs we take as we age, the better we will be physically and mentally.

As you age, you may want to consider changing healthcare providers. This can be hard for some people who are "used to" their doctor. However, you may want to switch to a doctor who understands slow medicine and all the nuances of aging. Often you can find a doctor in a regional nonprofit community health care system or a "concierge" practice that limit the number of patients they see so they can spend much more quality time with you at each appointment.

In addition to the physical changes we experience as we age, to thrive we also must accept the emotional losses we face. We may grieve the loss of our youth, our strength, or intellectual prowess. It's okay to grieve the loss of your own 20-something body. It helps you accept your current aging body. Although retirement offers freedom from the career grind, we may grieve the loss of our worklife identity. We also grieve the loss of beloved family members, friends, and pets. Grieving is normal, natural, and absolutely necessary.

By accepting that you are aging, you actually will age with a better attitude. Attitude may not be everything, but it helps a lot! You are not helpless to the sands of time. According to the Harvard School of Medicine, to maintain an independent and heathy lifestyle longer, there are five important factors you have control over. To thrive while aging:

1. Quit smoking. (Smoking increases the likelihood of being admitted to a nursing home by 56%.)

2. Get moving/Stay active. (Activity, both physical and mental, are your friends.)

3. Maintain a healthy weight.

4. Control your blood pressure.

5. Notice your fatigue.

If you are doing all of the above to keep yourself active and healthy and still find yourself frequently fatigued, tell your doctor! Heart disease, blood clots in the lungs or legs and other serious conditions may develop slowly. If you simply chalk up increasing fatigue to aging, those serious but treatable conditions continue to go undetected until they become an emergent medical crisis.

Recognizing your inevitable aging is part of living well. If you deny you are aging, then you also may deny that inevitably you will die. But honestly we all know we cannot escape death. We can live well, and we can die well. That is the whole point of this book—helping you consciously plan for the end of your life.

Planning ahead helps ensure that you experience a fulfilling life, and a death that is as peaceful, comfortable, and as comforting as possible for you and all those you leave behind.

Now are you ready to think about that?

Normal Aging Checklist

- Embrace your aging as a beautiful, normal and natural process
- Recognize normal age changes—physical, mental, and emotional
- Stay active and engaged in your family, community, and your special interests
- Adapt your activity and lifestyle according to your normal age changes and condition
- Prepare for the physical and emotional losses that occur as we age
- Consider "slow medicine" as aging continues:
  - Chose a doctor knowledgeable in aging who understands your goals of care
  - Tell your doctor about any increased fatigue, pain, weight changes, depression, loneliness
  - Keep medications to a minimum and frequently review medications with your doctor or pharmacist
  - Ask questions about every medication or medical test your doctor discusses and together decide what is best for you and your life goals
  - Have a family member or trusted friend accompany you to healthcare appointments to listen and corroborate what you think you hear during discussions with your doctor. Four ears and eyes are better than two when discussing serious health concerns.

Be brave enough to start a conversation that matters.
Dau Voire

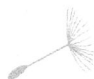

CHAPTER 2

PLAN YOUR CARE IN ADVANCE

We only die once.....so we have no experience doing it. And we don't like to think about it. But it's time.

Most of us, when asked about death, want to be upright one minute and in eternal peace the next. We don't want the prolonged discomfort of a lengthy terminal illness or loss of physical or mental capacity. Sudden unexpected death may seem to be a blessing, but it is shocking to those left behind, and frankly, not the norm. As much as "gone-in-an-instant" sounds preferable, it is more likely that most of us will experience a slow decline as we age and a lingering dying process.

Some people may experience a serious illness that brings a sudden sharp deterioration, but many will wane in a gradual stair-step fashion. We go along, living our life, perhaps fit and healthy for decades, until an illness occurs. We bounce back from that illness but not quite to the level we were before. As we age, those stair steps become more frequent and we keep marking new baselines of what is now our new normal health. Finally we are faced with an illness that is not curable but treatable. We may already have several other chronic illnesses that we cope with as well. So the reality is that death is usually not sudden. And it can be planned for.

The majority of people when polled about the end of life say they want to die peacefully at home, surrounded by family and friends. However, only a small percentage actually do die at home. Who do you know who has done so? Or instead, have you witnessed friends and family die in the hospital (or nursing/rehab facility) after a prolonged time?

There are several reasons people do not die according to their wishes. Number one, they don't make their wishes known or write them down or talk about what they want with those they love. There is no harm in reminding your family what you want should an emergency arrive. You might even have a Do Not Resuscitate (DNR) order on file and an Advanced Directive written, but still could find yourself hospitalized in an emergency situation without those essential documents. A medical crisis can cause chaos. And emotions. You may not be in the state of mind or physically able to voice your wishes. Do those closest to you know what you want?

I vividly recall a patient, Roxanne, a middle-aged woman with end-stage heart disease struggling to breathe, eyes wide, gasping for each breath. Roxanne had signed her DNR orders when she was admitted. But at the moment of her breathing crisis, with her mother by her bedside, the young resident asked Roxanne if she wanted to change her decision and have full heroic measures. Roxanne could not answer but her mother, panicked by seeing her daughter's struggle, said, "Yes! Do everything you can!" At that, Roxanne shook her head violently, signaling that she did not want heroics. I asked the resident if he would order morphine to ease her breathing. Thankfully, he agreed. Instead of subjecting Roxanne to a full code that would not have been successful, given her end-stage disease, the medication helped her breathe easier and she became calm.

Even when hospice is involved, sometimes family members panic. They call 911 when they were supposed to call the hospice team. Emergency responders come and take the patient to the hospital thus reintroducing the patient to acute intensive care when that person had planned to die peacefully at home. How can we prevent this from happening? How can we have our death be according to our wishes? We must fully contemplate our aging, and we must address our inevitable death. Now.

The best time to think about the type of care you want at the end of life is while you are healthy, with all of your faculties. By doing so, you make important care decisions based on what you deem most important in life, and what you need to feel satisfied with your quality of life when you are ill. It may be hard to think about your death while you are healthy, but it is much more difficult to make clear decisions in the midst of a life-limiting illness or emergency.

As a nation of planners, it's ironic that we plan everything, except for how we want to die. We plan little things and big things...from our children's playdates, to our careers, our vacations, our retirements, our weekend golf games, our weekly menus, our haircuts.... We plan a lot. We even plan for life insurance so in the event of our death, our family is taken care of financially. But we do not plan how we want to live as we face our inescapable death. As a society we do not talk easily and openly about death. Such conversation is still seen as "morbid" and depressing. But that need not be the case. We joke that the only two constants in life are death and taxes, and we plan for our taxes, but we do not plan for our own death.

Today healthy lifestyles and advances in medicine have made living well into our 70's and 80's the norm. Indeed, the fastest growing group in the U.S. are those over age 85. The number of people living to age 100 rose 44% between 2000 and 2014. Yes, we are living longer. But not forever.

The consequences of not planning for our eventual old age, debilitation, and unavoidable death often results in healthcare situations we would not choose for ourselves. Do you want cardiopulmonary resuscitation and ventilator-assisted breathing if you are already paralyzed and rendered speechless by multiple previous strokes? Do you want a feeding tube directly into your stomach when you are in advanced stages of dementia and no longer capable of swallowing? There are endless scenarios. Have you thought about what YOU want?

Families often will beseech doctors and nurses to "do something." Medical professionals have the training, dedication, and deep desire to indeed do something. With today's technological healthcare advances we can do almost anything to keep the physical body going.

We can keep your heart beating and your lungs functioning mechanically. However, by doing so, we may render you speechless, unable to function, or engage in any way with your loved ones. It's time for everyone to be clear-eyed and conscious of the fact that "doing something" may only extend physical existence, and does not mean prolonging a life of quality, of restored energy, of thriving. Many times, the things done in the name of healthcare merely prolong the dying process.

Healthcare professionals are quick to address your physical body's circumstance but may fail to address your individual mental, emotional, and spiritual needs or desires. Upon graduation from medical school and nursing school, new physicians and nurses pledge a solemn vow to uphold specific ethical standards, including to protect the people we serve from all harm or injustice. The physician's Hippocratic Oath and the nurse's Nightingale Pledge have undergone many revisions since ancient days but the essence of the vows remain the same—our dedication to serve people battling illness to the best of our ability.

As medical science has advanced, we are able to do so much more to sustain life. New technologies, surgical procedures, and a multitude of new drugs are available. But using them to continue to treat an incurable, terminal illness is not fully honoring those vows to protect our patients from harm. By continuing to offer acute care measures and asking you as a patient to decide without fully informing you of the likely actual effects of the procedure or drug, we simply prolong your dying without the comforts that hospice and palliative care provide. Just because we can do those procedures or use those new drugs does not necessarily mean we should use them.

To Code or Not to Code? That is the Question

Long before an accident occurs or a life-threatening illness strikes, it is wise to contemplate the kind of care you want to receive. What do you want to happen should your heart stop beating or your breathing stops?

That question should not be posed to you when you are in the Emergency Room. The ER is not the place or time to have an in-depth, contemplative discussion of the pros and cons of life-sustaining treatment. Health care providers often call such intervention "heroic measures." Indeed, it does take heroic effort to restart a failed heart and restore breathing. First, someone has to recognize you are experiencing a life-threatening event. Then emergency responders need to provide artificial breathing and chest compressions to restart your heart and your breathing. All these activities need to take place within 4-6 minutes of the initial event before your brain cells begin to die. With each passing minute with no heartbeat or breathing, you risk "living" a life of permanent disability or not waking at all, being trapped in what health professionals call a "permanent vegetative state." Television medical dramas often show emergency measures being used that magically restore the actor patient to full health in the course of the 60-minute drama. In real life however, those heroic measures do not often restore the person to full, robust health and certainly not immediately.

Cardiopulmonary Resuscitation (CPR)
Cardiopulmonary resuscitation (CPR) measures range from simple mouth-to-mouth breathing and chest compressions to use of an automated electronic defibrillator

(AED) to shock the heart into a normal rhythm, along with automatic ventilation by inserting breathing tubes through the trachea, and life-sustaining medications. In 1960 the American Heart Association (AHA) developed the original CPR program to acquaint doctors with closed chest compressions to restart hearts during cardiac operations. That first program led to standardized training programs and performance standards for the general public. According to the AHA, "bystander CPR" in the general public is effective; those who receive CPR by trained bystanders are three times more likely to survive than those who do not have CPR for sudden cardiac arrest. However the early program was intended primarily to help victims of sudden cardiac arrest such as in heart attack, electrocution or drowning. CPR was not intended to be what it has become—a universal method of resuscitation for everyone, regardless of age or condition. Since the mid-1970s, CPR has become the standard for healthcare professionals in any healthcare setting to perform on any patient who does not have a "Do Not Resuscitate" order. That need not be the case.

Performing CPR on a patient already hospitalized for life-threatening conditions or illness, especially an older patient, rarely restores the person to full physical and mental function. Chest compressions on elderly patients with osteoporosis (brittle bones) can result in what we call a "flailed chest," in which the bones in the rib cage fracture under the force needed to successfully restore the heartbeat. Such rib fractures can further complicate the life-threatening event by lacerating the liver. The medical team may successfully restore the patient's heart rhythm and breathing, but sustaining the heartbeat and breathing may require the patient to be connected to a ventilator either temporarily or long-term. Long-term ventilator-dependence may damage airways or cause internal bleeding. Ventilators are effective in maintaining breathing but the tracheal tube is intensely uncomfortable, so much so that often the patient must be sedated or restrained so they do not pull the tracheal tube out and do not fight against the ventilator rhythm. When normal secretions accumulate in the tracheal tube, the tube must be suctioned or the person chokes. Suctioning is uncomfortable and can be frightening. Lack of oxygen through the patient's body while the heart is not beating and the patient is not breathing may result in either loss of physical function or brain damage or both. In such cases, CPR may simply result in complicating and prolonging the dying process.

As a nursing student, I was drawn to general medicine and oncology over other areas of healthcare. I loved getting to know and care for "my" patients, who were often older and more frail. Their life stories impressed and inspired me to provide care to them as if they were my parents or grandparents. But I always loathed hearing the "Code" announcement, fearing that aggressive and frantic exercise of chest compressions and resuscitation would add to my patients' suffering.

I have cared for many patients who initially survived CPR but were not restored to anything close to their previous health or active lives. Resuscitation was never intended to be done for every hospitalized patient without regard for their underlying condition leading to that cardiac or respiratory arrest.

The actual statistics of CPR survival are sobering. According to a 2010 article in The Hospitalist, hospitalized patients overestimate their chance of surviving cardiac arrest by 60%, when in reality only about 17% of all hospitalized patients who have heroic measures of CPR survive to be discharged. And only about 6% of older hospitalized patients with multiple medical problems or who cannot live independently survive heroic measures to be discharged.

Lucy was a 75-year-old patient who had been in a coma after receiving CPR for a heart attack at age 62. At the time of her heart attack, she had not made any decisions about her future health, or her death. In the ensuring thirteen years, Lucy had gained more than sixty pounds from the tube feedings with no ability to move or burn those calories. Her family was unwilling to make the decision to stop the tube feedings or remove her from the ventilator. Lucy died of "drowning" when her feeding tube had become dislodged from her esophagus and her liquid meal went down her trachea into her lungs. Lucy's end of life could have been drastically different.

Do Not Resuscitate (DNR)

Do Not Resuscitate (DNR) is a doctor's order that instructs health care providers about your wishes to not have CPR initiated in an emergency if your heart stops beating or you stop breathing. The DNR is a medical form signed by your physician that is best completed in advance of a serious health condition. It requires you to have a frank discussion with your doctor about your wishes. Both you and your doctor keep a copy of your DNR; one in your medical chart in your doctor's office and one for you to show any healthcare provider or emergency responder who visits your home. You can also share copies with your family so they know your wishes, too. Take your DNR form with you if you are hospitalized. The DNR pertains only to CPR and does not address other healthcare treatment such as pain control, other medications, nutrition or fluids. DNR is accepted in every state in the US and in use in every hospital and healthcare setting.

This decision of Do Not Resuscitate is critical. It may not be easy to think about tragic circumstances befalling you, but the situation becomes much more tragic if you do not address it ahead of time. Take the time now to have these important discussions with your doctor and to share your end-of-life choices with your family.

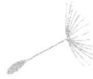

*I have an advance directive, not because I have a serious
illness, but because I have a family.*
Dr. Ira Byock

CHAPTER 3

ADVANCE DIRECTIVES

Mary Lou, age 88, had lived fifteen years with ever-advancing dementia. Her daughter had cared for her at home for years. When the dementia caused increasing agitation, Mary Lou was moved to a memory unit of a nearby beautiful assisted living residence and her daughter and friends visited daily. Despite Mary Lou's poor health and very advanced dementia, hospice services were not initiated nor her wishes detailed. When Mary Lou suffered an intestinal tear, she was taken to the hospital for surgical repair. Her dementia was complicated by delirium after surgery. Terrified and agitated, she required deep sedation to keep her calm and safe from doing herself harm even in her weakened state. She succumbed to the dementia and post-op complications in the hospital a week after surgery. Had detailed advanced directives been in place as well as hospice services, she would not have suffered the physical trauma and emotional terror she experienced as a surgical patient in an unfamiliar, frightening setting.

An Advance Directive is a form you complete (or create yourself) in which you:

1. Appoint another person to make health care decisions for you if or when you lose the capacity to make your own healthcare decisions. This appointment is typically referred to as your "healthcare durable power of attorney" or "healthcare proxy."
2. Provide guidance for making healthcare decisions at the end of life, usually referred to as a "living will."

The advance directive or "living will" is written direction from you in anticipation of you becoming a patient with a life-threatening illness. It is a legal form, approved by each state legislature and signed by a lawyer. It is not a medical order like the DNR.

An advance directive does not have to be complicated. You can create your own by simply writing the kind of healthcare you want—or do not want—to receive. You can also choose to complete a computerized form that includes all the healthcare parameters recognized by your state of residence. Whatever way you choose to create your advance directive, make sure it meets your state's requirements.

Once you have written your advance directive, have your lawyer review it to confirm your directives are understood exactly as you intend. When you are satisfied it is as you wish, have your advance directives notarized and give copies to your family and your doctor.

You may designate a family member, close friend or neighbor to serve as Durable Power of Attorney for Health Care or Health Care Proxy. This person is given authority to make any healthcare decision for you if you cannot make decisions for yourself. Your healthcare power of attorney should know you well enough to be secure in making decisions as you would make if you had the ability to do so.

When I was an eldercare manager, one of my clients, Maria, was a 38-year-old woman who had been in a serious car accident five years previously while on vacation in Mexico. She did not have signed advance directives at the time of the accident. Maria had sustained severe head trauma when the cab she was in crashed into a concrete abutment. The medical clinic in the small Mexican village where she was first taken was not equipped to provide the intense neurological care she required. Maria survived her transfer to the U.S. for additional care but "coded" after suffering a series of seizures in the course of her initial treatment. Despite her medical team showing her family that Maria had no discernible brain activity, they could not agree on the decision for "Do Not Resuscitate" orders. To the best of my knowledge she remains in a permanent vegetative state today.

Because of my nursing career, and my passion on this topic, I am sure you are not surprised to learn that I have fully considered the kind of care I wish to receive as I age and when I face an illness that cannot be cured. Currently I'm healthy and active, in my late sixties. I see my concierge physician once a year for a 90-minute physical exam and comprehensive wellness profile. I have an annual mammogram and a screening colonoscopy every three years given my family history of colon cancer and my own history of colon polyps. Although I deeply enjoy my current health, I have discussed my wishes for end-of-life care with my physician and have signed Do Not Resuscitate orders that are currently in my medical chart and a copy at home. I have also designated my healthcare power of attorney and have signed a detailed "living will" on file with my attorney, and have a copy at home. My healthcare power of attorney is also my financial power of attorney. My husband and adult children know my end-of-life wishes, probably in far greater detail than they really want to know at this point in my life. But for years I have stressed to them how important it is to plan ahead. And how much of their burden of care will be relieved by my prior planning. Since I am currently in good health, the copies of my advanced directives are filed in the desk in our study, and everyone knows this.

Should I become ill with a life-limiting illness, the DNR will be posted prominently over my bed so rescue personnel will be fully informed of my healthcare decisions even if I am unable to speak to confirm my wishes.

My husband's diagnosis of a potentially life-limiting illness propelled me into a higher gear of healthcare planning for him and for myself. Glenn was diagnosed with indolent follicular Non-Hodgkin lymphoma, a type of lymphoma that is imminently treatable but not generally curable. Glenn opted for the most aggressive treatment available at the time. He had much to live for, including the weddings of our son and daughter scheduled in the spring and summer following his four-month treatment. But his illness served as another "wake-up" call that Life is fleeting. We took that opportunity to "put our estate in order" both in healthcare and financial plans. Remarkably, Glenn has enjoyed a complete, sustained remission for ten years. While his health has been stable, we have frequently revisited our advance directives, living wills, and chosen proxies to make sure all of us know each other's wishes.

These decisions call into play your values. Is it most important to you to use every means available to stay alive, no matter the cost? Or do you choose to simply "let it be" and not to prolong the dying process by artificial means? Making these decisions ahead of the time frees you from having to make decisions when you are in the midst of a health crisis. Your advance planning is also an immeasurable gift to those you love. By deciding what you want and communicating your wishes to them, you take the burden of care off their shoulders. Make your own decisions about healthcare well in advance, and inform your loved ones of your wishes. Doing so helps eliminates guilt or regret or any prism of emotions they would feel if they had to make decisions for you.

Fully consider the responsibility you are asking of your chosen healthcare proxy. They must be completely willing and emotionally capable to carry out your wishes when you are unable to do so for yourself. Husbands and wives, brothers and sisters, sons and daughters may agree initially before the health crisis to carry out your wishes but may balk when the actual situation requires their action. Talk about these possibilities now. If you are living alone and away from immediate family members, you may want to consider asking a trusted friend to serve as your healthcare proxy. In any case, keep having the conversation about your wishes with the person you choose as your healthcare proxy to make sure they remain entirely committed to carrying out your wishes. And continue the conversation with all your loved ones to be sure they are fully aware of what is most important to you in your life and in your death.

Patty's mom, Elsie, had a history of chronic obstructive pulmonary disease (COPD) that had been manageable with medications and supplemental oxygen.

However, when Elsie developed pneumonia, her respiratory status was severely compromised and she required hospital care. The medical team recommended aiding her breathing through intubation and short-term ventilator use, to which Elsie agreed. But her pneumonia did not respond to the intravenous antibiotics. She had to continue to endure ventilator breathing while other antibiotics were tried. Weeks went by and Elsie's condition did not improve. The tube in her trachea prevented her from speaking, but Elsie communicated very well with her facial expressions and hand squeezes. Elsie made it clear she had had enough when after a long gaze at her daughter, and a tight hand grip, Elsie flung Patty's hand aside as if to say, "I'm done!" Patty asked the medical team to discontinue the ventilator, but continue the intravenous fluids and oxygen. Early the following morning, Elsie died peacefully, surrounded by Patty and her family.

As an eldercare manager, one of my most important responsibilities was to establish my clients' end-of-life wishes, and help them complete their advance directives, including their DNR orders with their physician. Those important forms were stored in a bright red folder, along with their insurance information, list of medications, phone numbers of healthcare providers, pharmacies, and family members. The folder was prominently displayed on the front of the refrigerator in easy reach for family and healthcare providers.

In an ideal world, all adults, regardless of health status, would have signed Advance Directives available so spouses and family members know how to proceed in the event of a medical emergency. Advance Directives are often included in estate planning and are also available in most healthcare settings. Today there are many different forms available through myriad organizations.

The idea of an advanced directive may feel daunting in and of itself, but as I will keep stating, end of life decisions should not be made at the end of life. The fact that you are reading this book means you are ready to prepare your wishes. There are a wide array of forms and formats to choose from when completing the paperwork. To make the documentation process easier for you, I have included two of my favorite options.

Years ago when I sought for myself an easy, readable format to express what I wanted to experience during my end of life, I discovered Five Wishes. When I worked as an eldercare manager, I was trained in the Physician Orders for Life Sustaining Treatment (POLST) Paradigm process to help my elder clients and their families.

Whatever form you choose, take the time NOW to discuss and write down your care goals so your family and health care team can do what you want for your life and death. Remember both of these advance directives are intended for those who are diagnosed with an illness that cannot be cured, yet it's always a good idea to have the talks with your family to make your preferences known no matter what you may face at end of life.

Five Wishes (https://fivewishes.org)

The nonprofit organization Aging with Dignity created and trademarked the "Five Wishes" living will form to document a person's physical, emotional, and spiritual needs when facing a life-limiting illness. Jim Tomey, one of the organization founders, had lived and worked closely with Mother Theresa in a hospice she founded in Washington, D.C. He was inspired by that experience to help patients and families plan ahead and created the Five Wishes process in 1998.

Five Wishes is written in plain language, is easy to read and complete, and encompasses legal and medical requirements as well as physical, emotional, and spiritual comforts.

The Five Wishes form includes:

- Whom you wish to be your healthcare proxy or healthcare durable power of attorney
- What medical treatment you wish or do not wish to have
- What level of physical, emotional, and spiritual comfort you wish to have
- How you wish others will treat you so your dignity is maintained
- What you wish your loved ones to know

Five Wishes was written with the help of the American Bar Association's Commission on Law & Aging. It meets the legal requirements of advance planning in 42 states and the District of Columbia and is widely used in all 50 states. If you live in one of the following states—Indiana, Kansas, Michigan, New Hampshire, Ohio, Oregon, Texas, Wyoming—you are required to complete specific additional forms. No matter where you live, you can still use Five Wishes to help guide the conversation. The Five Wishes form is available in 27 languages and Braille. You can obtain the form from your attorney or online. The form is easily updated or changed, depending on your evolving needs and desires.

At the center of Five Wishes is the emphasis on having conversations about what specific type of care you want. As they state on their website, "it's more than just a document. Five Wishes is a complete approach to discussing and documenting your care and comfort choices." Get more information at https://agingwithdignity.org and https://fivewishes.org.

Physician's Orders for Life-Sustaining Treatment (POLST) Paradigm (https://polst.org)

Similar to Five Wishes, the Physician's Order for Life-Sustaining Treatment (POLST) is a process designed to improve patient care by creating a portable medical form that records a patient's treatment wishes.

Begun in Oregon in 1991, POLST is available in many states across the country. Some states have shortened the title from POLST to POST, changing the term "life-sustaining" to "scope." Others have implemented MOST programs, changing "physician" to "medical." Despite the word changes, POLST, POST, and MOST are all identical in their intent to help you make the difficult treatment decisions when faced with life-limiting illness or advanced, frail age.

Like Five Wishes and other advance planning tools, POLST involves a series of crucial conversations between you and your family, your doctor, nurse practitioner or physician assistant. These conversations help you specify your goals of care, what kind of care you want and how much care you want given your current diagnosis, prognosis, and various treatment options.

Unlike the Advanced Directives that all adults should have regardless of their health status, the POLST decision-making conversations and resulting doctors' orders are intended for people who are at risk of having an emergent life threatening event because they already have a serious life-limiting medical condition that cannot be cured or they have advanced frailty due to age or dementia.

Examples of medical conditions that pose a threat of a medical emergent event include:

1. Severe heart disease

2. Metastatic cancer or malignant brain tumor

3. Advanced lung disease

4. Advanced neurodegenerative disease (dementia, Parkinson's, Amyotrophic Lateral Sclerosis (ALS), Multiple Sclerosis.

5. Advanced frailty (advanced chronic disease and/or advanced age with significant weight loss and functional decline)

The POLST form clearly states the specific medical orders that apply only to you regarding the medical treatments you would want to receive.

The POLST form does not replace the Advance Directives of healthcare proxy but is a helpful adjunct. The two documents work together to clearly communicate your specific medical treatment wishes in the event of a medical emergency after you have been diagnosed with a life-limiting illness. The important difference between Advance Directives and POLST orders is that advanced directives are legal forms, written by a lawyer, and POLST is a set of medical orders, signed by your physician.

Like the DNR, the POLST form is voluntary; it is your choice whether you want one or not. The POLST lets the emergency medical service (EMS) team know whether or not you want CPR. Remember that the DNR

(Do Not Resuscitate) order only applies when you do not have a pulse, are not breathing, or unresponsive. The POLST provides much more information to the EMS team including whether you want:

1. Full treatment—hospitalization and all treatment options available, including use of a ventilator for breathing.

2. Limited treatment—hospitalization for basic treatment (antibiotics, stabilization) but not including intensive care.

3. Comfort care only—no hospitalization; pain control and symptom management at home or wherever you are living.

The POLST form is a double-sided single sheet of brightly colored (generally neon pink, yellow, or green) card stock. POLST is designed to be: Doctor's Orders—specifically directing what you should receive and not receive in a hospital or healthcare setting; and Portable—easy to grab in an emergency.

POLST discussions and the POLST form can help you and your family make the hard decisions when faced with a life-limiting illness, and most importantly, your own goals of care. These conversations will help you, your doctor, and your family do the important advanced planning so everyone is "on the same page" regarding your treatment and care wishes.

The conversations that the POLST paradigm generate include:

1. Hospitalization—When faced with a life-limiting illness or in advanced frailty, either at home or living in a senior residence such as a nursing home, should you be hospitalized or simply receive comfort care? Is it time to shift from curative care to comfort care? What are your goals of treatment if you cannot be cured and curative treatment does not exist?

2. Resuscitation or Artificial Ventilation—Restarting the heart of a frail elderly person may not bring the person back to their previous baseline. We have already discussed resuscitation in the previous chapter so you understand the risks. When faced with a life-limiting illness or in advanced frailty, do you want resuscitation? To receive artificial ventilation?

3. Artificial nutrition (feeding tubes or parenteral nutrition)—Do you want to be fed by artificial means if you can no longer take in food? (FYI, nasogastric tubes can become dislodged from the esophagus. When that happens the liquid meal can be aspirated into the lungs causing aspiration pneumonia or actual respiratory arrest due to drowning. And of course we know that artificial feeding in advanced dementia does not cure the dementia. It simply prolongs the dying process.)

4. Intravenous hydration—Do you wish to be hydrated via intravenous tubes if you can no longer sip water? (Please know that hydrating tumors in end stage cancer results in more discomfort and pain. In the natural world, animals cease drinking and eating as the end of life nears.)

5. Use of antibiotics—What do you wish for your end of life? (Similar to artificial hydration, use of antibiotics can prolong the dying process. Prior to wide-spread availability and use of antibiotics, pneumonia was referred to as "the old man's friend" since the condition caused the sufferer to lapse into unconsciousness and peacefully slip away in their sleep. Pneumonia was considered to provide a dignified end to a person's suffering.)

6. Renal or peritoneal dialysis—When your kidneys start shutting down, what do you want done for you? (When kidneys fail, the toxins that would normally be dispelled in urine build up in the body. Dialysis removes the toxins but doing so at the end of life can simply prolong death, without adding quality to the remaining life. Dialysis must be done frequently to keep the toxins from accumulating. Depending on the type of dialysis, you would need to be able to travel to a dialysis center up to three times a week or more or

be able to have the procedure done at home, either by yourself or someone trained to do it properly.)

As you can see, the POLST form gets you thinking about the harsh realities you face during end of life care.

The POLST form is kept by you at home (or with you in the hospital, or wherever you are living). Your doctor or health care provider also keeps a copy in your medical records. The POLST form is meant to be portable. For easy access at home, put the POLST form on your refrigerator, or on your medicine cabinet, or clearly visible near your bed. Remind your family and friends that you have a POLST so they can tell emergency medical staff to look for it. Provide a copy to your chosen durable power of attorney for healthcare (or healthcare proxy). Keep a copy in your purse or wallet when you are traveling so emergency medical staff can find it.

Like the DNR and other Advance Directives, POLST forms were created to be easily revised. If your medical condition changes or your goals of care change, all you have to do is talk with your doctor, nurse practitioner, or physician assistant so they can update the POLST form. If you decide you no longer want a POLST form in place, your health care provider can easily void the document. Instructions on how to void are included on the form.

Currently the POLST program is in full use in twelve states and is being implemented in 24 more states.

Remember that the POLST is portable medical orders and thus must be signed by your healthcare provider to be valid. For more information, go to https://polst.org.

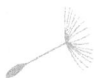

It is up to YOU to make these decisions NOW.

As always, communication is the key to making these tough decisions for yourself and for your family. Together with your family and your physician, you determine the specific care you want and how you want that care to be delivered. Once you make these decisions, make sure you sign the required legal and healthcare forms and keep them handy!

All of your preparation will not be effective if the forms are filed away and are not accessible at the time of an unexpected health crisis.

As time goes on, you may reconsider some of the decisions you make today. Make sure you keep your loved ones informed of any changes in your wishes. The time you put in now contemplating the end of your life is time well spent. Always remember that love's last act is for those you cherish as well as yourself.

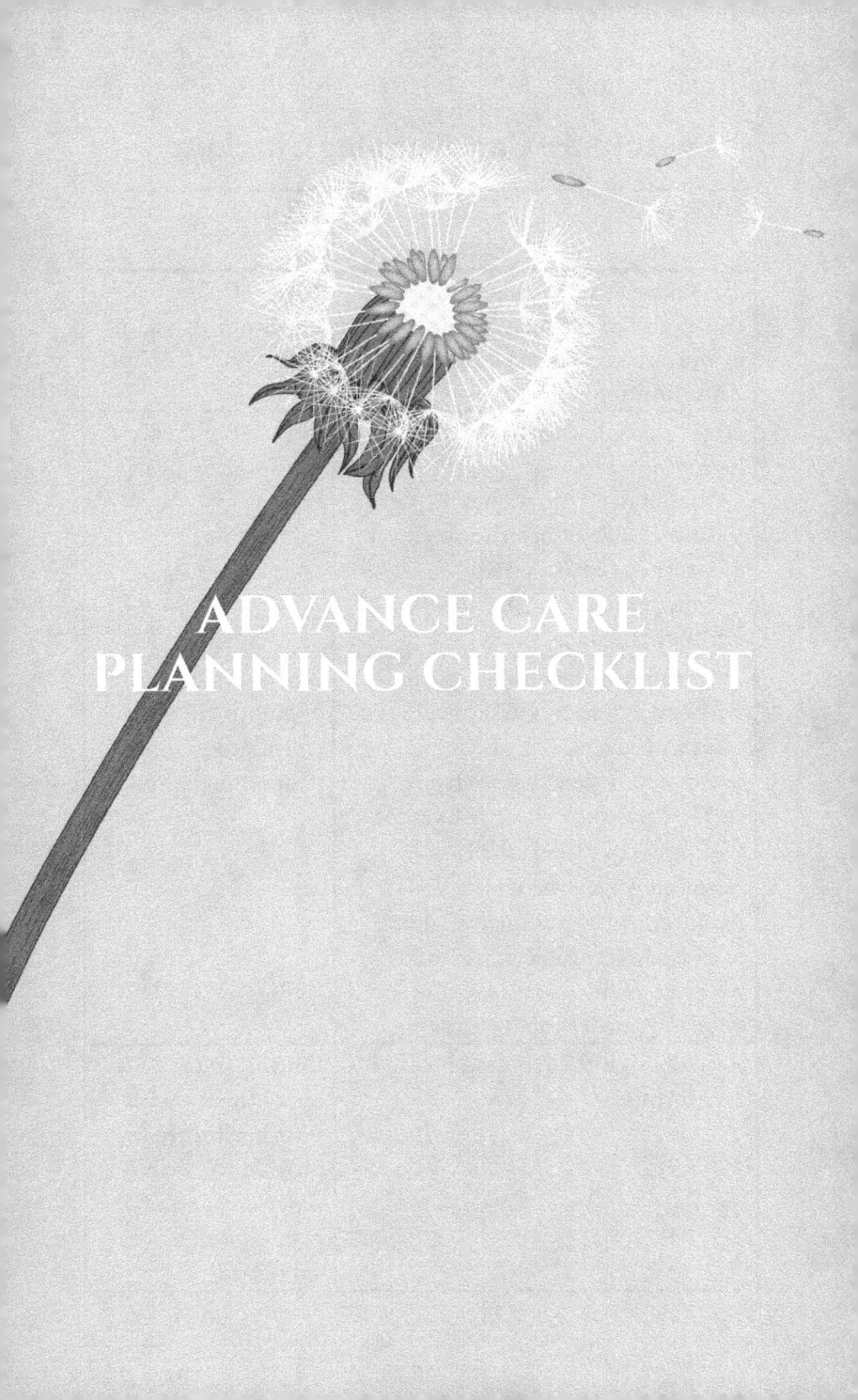

ADVANCE CARE PLANNING CHECKLIST

Advance Care Planning Checklist

What to Do	When
Take time to fully consider the type and extent of medical care you want as you age and when you are facing a life-limiting illness.	Now—Before a life-limiting health crisis
Begin the conversation with your loved ones. Discuss: —Your end-of-life wishes —Your choice of healthcare power of attorney (health proxy) —Your choice of financial power of attorney (financial proxy)	Now—Before a life-limiting health crisis
Talk with your doctor about the type and extent of medical care you want as you age. Ask about signing: —Advance Directives such as — Do Not Resuscitate (DNR) or — Physician Orders for Life Sustaining Treatment) (POLST) Keep copies of your medical directives easily accessible at home so when a health crisis arises, your loved ones and proxies can have them.	Now—Make an appointment for a consultation or at your annual physical
Actually sign the required healthcare form(s)	During your appointment with your healthcare provider or within a week or two of your consultation appointment

What to Do	When
Talk with your lawyer about signing: —A Living Will —Power of Attorney for Healthcare —Power of Attorney for Finances	Now—Make an office or phone appointment
Actually sign the required legal form(s)	During your office visit with your lawyer or mail your signed forms to your lawyer within a week or two following your appointment
Provide a copy of your Advance Directives, including your Living Will to your chosen Power of Attorney for Healthcare (Health-care proxy)	As soon as you have copies of the required signed forms available to share
Provide a copy of estate planning, Last Will and Testament, your Living Will and Advance Directives to your chosen Financial Power of Attorney	As soon as you have copies of the required signed forms available to share
Continue to review your legal and healthcare forms and update your health and legal forms as you need.	When your health is stable, review every six months. When your health changes, review more often to ensure you receive the care you desire

Physician's Orders for Life-Sustaining Treatment (POLST) by State (https://polst.org/programs-in-your-state/)

California (https://capolst.org/polst-for-patients-loved-ones)

Florida (https://polstfl.org)

Georgia (www.gapolst.org)

Maine (https://www.mainehospicecouncil.org/index.php/home/polst-physician-orders-for-life-sustaining-treatment)

Montana (b.bsd.dli.mt.gov/license/bsd_boards/med_board/polst.asp)

New Hampshire (https://www.healthynh.com/provider-orders-for-life-sustaining-treatment-polst.html)

North Dakota (www.honoringchoicesnd.org/polst)

Washington (https://wsma.org/POLST)

Wisconsin (www.gundersenhealth.org/advance-care/resources)

Other Names for POLST programs by State

AZPOLST Arizona Provider Orders for Life-Sustaining Treatment (https://azpolst.org)

DMOST Delaware Medical Orders for Scope of Treatment (delawaremost.org)

IPOST Iowa Physicians Orders for Scope of Treatment (www.ihconline.org/aspx/initiatives/ipost.aspx)

LaPOST Louisiana Physician Order for Scope of Treatment (https://lhcqf.org/lapost)

MOLST (Medical Orders for Life-Sustaining Treatment)

Connecticut (portal.ct.gov/DPH/Medical-Orders-for-Life-Sustaining-Treatment-MOLST/MOLST)

Maryland (marylandmolst.org/index.html)

Massachusetts (https://www.molst-ma.org)

New York (https://molst.org)

Rhode Island (https://healthcentricadvisors.org/myccv/pt)

MOST (Medical Orders for Scope of Treatment)

Colorado (https://www.civhc.org/programs-and-services/
advance-care-planning)

District of Columbia (https://dchealth.dc.gov/most)

Kentucky (https://www.kymost.org)

New Mexico (http://www.nmmost.org)

North Carolina (compassionatecarenc.org)

South Dakota (https://sdaho.org/most)

Texas (www.northtexasrespectingchoices.com/m-o-s-t)

OkPOLST (Oklahoma Physician Orders for Life-Sustaining Treatment)

Oklahoma (https://www.practicalbioethics.org/programs/
transportable-physician-orders-for-patient-preferences)

PAPOLST (Pennsylvania Orders for Life-Sustaining Treatment)

Pennsylvania (www.papolst.org)

POST (Physician Orders for Scope of Treatment)

Idaho (https://sos.idaho.gov/HCDRSearch/search.aspx)

Indiana (www.indianapost.org)

South Carolina (https://www.scdhec.gov/physician-orders-
scope-treatment-post)

Tennessee (endoflifecaretn.org)

Virginia (www.virginiapost.org)

West Virginia (wvendoflife.org/home)

POLST (Practitioner Orders for Life-Sustaining Treatment)

Illinois (www.polstil.org)

New Jersey (www.njha.com/polst)

POLST (Provider Orders for Life-Sustaining Treatment)

Hawaii (http://www.kokuamau.org)

Minnesota (http://www.mnmed.org/advocacy/improving-health-of-minnesotans/POLST-Communications)

Nevada (www.nevadapolst.org)

Utah (https://bemsp.utah.gov/operations-and-response/ems-operations/advance-care-directives)

POLST (Portable Orders for Life-Sustaining Treatment)

Oregon (oregonpolst.org)

TPOPP (Transportable Physician Orders for Patient Preferences)

Kansas (https://www.practicalbioethics.org/programs/transportable-physician-orders-for-patient-preferences)

Missouri (https://www.practicalbioethics.org/programs/transportable-physician-orders-for-patient-preferences)

WyoPOLST (Providers Orders for Life Sustaining Treatment)

Wyoming (https://www.wyomed.org/wyopolst)

Dying is neither a medical condition or a spiritual
condition. It is simply a human condition.
Frank Bennet, MD

CHAPTER 4

DYING—WE ALL DO IT

S ome will die suddenly. Others will die after a very
brief illness. And many (dare I say most) will experience a long, lingering decline before the final dying day
arrives. The 21st century advances in U.S. healthcare offer
us almost unlimited means to prolong life, yet despite
using every measure to thwart death, ultimately we will
die. Given that we can receive almost endless medical
treatment, how do we decide type and extent of medical
care in the face of terminal illness?

To help determine your goals, Hank Dunn, a long-
time hospice chaplain and author of Hard Choices for
Loving People, suggests asking yourself this query:

Do you expect your medical treatment to achieve:

- A complete cure of your illness?
- Preserve your functionality?
- Provide you peace through comfort care?

Many life-limiting illnesses can successfully be treated, if not cured. My husband has enjoyed a decade-long sustained, complete remission of his non-Hodgkin lymphoma. He continues to be satisfied living with the lingering after-effects of the harsh treatment he endured. But now that Glenn is in his seventh decade, he knows his treatment plan will be different should the lymphoma recur or he develops a second cancer or other illness.

When your illness cannot be completely cured, what trade-offs in your routine or lifestyle are you willing to make to continue living your life as best you can, given your health condition? Dr. Atul Gawande, Dr. Frank Bennet, of the Living Well/Dying Well initiative, and other end-of-life physicians agree that asking yourself such questions helps clarify what is most important for you. In doing so, your choices make it clear not only to you but also to your family and to your healthcare team, and helps maximize your comfort, peace and satisfaction as you face the end of life.

It is up to you whether you "fight to the death" or you choose less aggressive means to treat your illness as you approach your dying day. You need to think things through for yourself, and the expert physician authors provide two questions to guide your process:

What makes life meaningful to me?

Of course, the answer to that question is different for all and the answer may change during the course of a final illness.

When are the tradeoffs too great to want to remain alive?

The trade-offs each of us are willing to make are as diverse as the answer to the first question.

For instance, I am willing to accept using assistive devices such as a wheelchair, shower chair, and upright walker to continue as active a life as possible.

I also am a "foodie." I love to cook and entertain. The experience of sitting around the table, savoring favorite foods with family and friends delights me. So the option of getting my nutrition only in liquid form via a feeding tube down my throat or directly into my stomach is abhorrent to me. In my advance directives I clearly state I do not wish to sustain life through artificial nutrition or hydration.

These questions require deep pondering on your part. You will thank yourself when you face a serious illness, as you may feel at least somewhat prepared. Facing what may be the final illness is always a shock. But by taking time now, well before receiving a devastating diagnosis, to think about what makes life meaningful and how you want to fill your final days will help you adjust to the news. Moreover, this preparation will be a gift to those who love you. They will not have to wonder what you want, nor will they feel guilt or regrets by helping carry out your wishes.

The nonprofit organization Compassion and Choices offers a "My End-of-Life Decisions" advance planning booklet that includes a "values" worksheet of ranked items to help you decide what is most important to you. The booklet contains other questions to ask and discuss with your family, including:

- Would you want life-sustaining treatments no matter the circumstance, or do you believe that when there is no hope of recovery, natural death should be allowed?
- What basic functional abilities are important to you in order to feel you would want to continue living?
- Are there treatments you would definitely want, or definitely not want, if you were diagnosed with a non-curable illness?
- Do you have a particular doctor you want to direct your care?
- Is there anyone you do not want involved in your health care or end-of life decisions?

Palliative Care and Hospice Care May Prolong Life

The aim of palliative care (comfort care) is to manage symptoms to achieve optimum quality of life in any health condition. Comfort care is an important part of aggressive medical treatments for life-limiting illnesses. But comfort care is of tantamount importance in terminal illness and is the cornerstone of hospice care. Hospice care differs from palliative care in that hospice care is specifically designed for those who are expected to die of their illness within six months.

Hospice care is not intended to either prolong life nor hasten death. Hospice doctors, nurses, and care staff assist you by helping you maintain your dignity, control your pain, and provide you the personal comforts you desire from the day you are admitted to hospice service to the day you die.

There are occasions when someone deemed terminal enters hospice care and improves physically and psychosocially because of the comfort care they receive. When such improvement happens, hospice celebrates "graduation" from hospice care and the patient returns to primary care.

In 2010 the New England Journal of Medicine published the results of a randomized controlled trial of certain cancer patients who received palliative care early in the course of their illness. The patients had significant improvements in both their quality of life and mood. Compared with patients receiving standard care (without palliative care), patients receiving early palliative care also survived more than three months longer than those who had the most aggressive care.

Hospice care is most effective when care is initiated several months before death is imminent. Comfort care that improves our physical, emotional, and spiritual well-being allows us to live longer. Unfortunately, the decision to shift from aggressive or curative treatment to comfort care is often made too late, in many cases within days or hours of death. Although hospice care has been available in the United States for over 40 years, the National Hospice and Palliative Care Organization (NHPCO) reports that the majority of people who enter hospice care today do so less than three weeks before their death.

Waiting too long to choose hospice care when coping with terminal illness robs you of reaping the benefits that hospice care offers. My purpose in writing this book, my dear readers, is to urge you to choose the comfort care that hospice provides, not only for you, but also for your household. Hospice comfort care extends to the entire circle of your family and friends, providing a higher quality of life for all involved during your dying process. Hospice comfort care continues after your death for your family and friends as they grapple with their bereavement. Hospice staff provide the essential, invaluable physical, emotional, and spiritual support for you during your dying days and they continue to provide support for those you love by providing grief and bereavement counseling.

There is no greater final gift we can give, to ourselves and beloveds, than to orchestrate our peaceful, comfortable death. Dying, we all do it. Am I getting through to you?

Points to Ponder About How You Wish to Die

- Contemplate what abilities and activities mean the most to you in life.

- Consider what you must have in order to enjoy a meaningful life.

- Think about what you would accept when faced with a life-limiting illness and what would be unbearable to endure.

- Talk with your doctor, nurse practitioner, or physician assistant about the type of comfort care you want to receive during any illness, especially a final illness.

- Explore the hospice services currently available in your community or your likely location when you are at the end of life.

- Consider who you want and who you do not want as your caregiver(s) to support you during your final illness.

- Consider the changes that may need to be made in your current living situation when you need hospice services:

  - Do you want to remain at home or do you want to move to an in-patient hospice facility?

    - Can your needs be met by family or friends at home or is the burden of direct care too great for those available at home?

- If you remain at home, how can your surroundings be adapted to provide you with ultimate comfort, such as:

  - locating the hospital bed in a living room or other location rather than bedroom in order to remain at the center of your family?

  - having a bathroom conveniently located to your bed location for you or for your caregiver?

Death is not the opposite of life but a part of it.
Haruki Murakami

CHAPTER 5

THE HOSPICE WAY

As Dr. Byock says, "Hospice does not guarantee that dying will be easy, pretty, or fun," but hospice care does effectively relieve pain and the myriad distressing elements of a terminal illness. Those who have a life-ending illness can withstand much higher doses of pain relieving drugs than a healthy body would tolerate. To quote Dr. Byock, "the right dose is the dose that works" to relieve pain. Pain medication is most often provided on a scheduled, 'round-the-clock' basis. When a person is no longer able to swallow pills or liquid, pain medication is given by subcutaneous injection (a relatively painless injection in the connective tissue of the skin using a very small needle).

A common side effect of pain medication is sleepiness but that usually resolves in a few days' time, so you can be comfortable and still enjoy the company and conversation of friends and family who visit you. Though appetite usually diminishes greatly as death draws near, hospice staff encourage you to enjoy favorite foods and drink favorite beverages as you can, even if it is a mere bite or small sip. The "wisdom of the body" will eventually reveal itself by ceasing eating and drinking. That does not indicate starvation but simply the lack of need by the physical body for fluids or calories. The point of hospice comfort care is to address the physical and emotional effects of illness so you can experience the highest quality of life through to the end of life.

I intend to secure hospice services precisely so I can continue to enjoy the foods and drinks I love best. Eggs of any style will take center stage on my tray. I will drink my coffee latte-style, strong, hot, and loaded with whipped cream. I will savor high-quality milk chocolate without concern about calories. And I will toast the setting sun with a glass filled with Tangueray and tonic, topped off with a slice of lime.

Where is hospice care provided?
Hospice care is most often provided in your home—whether you live in an apartment, condo, single family home, or in a nursing home, assisted living facility, or other setting. Some hospice agencies also offer inpatient services in hospitals, freestanding hospice facilities, skilled nursing facilities, or assisted living residences.

Hospice services generally do not provide full time professional caregivers. Most often, your family or friends serve as caregivers with help from hospice doctors and nurses. A hospice physician will work with your primary physician to plan your care. A hospice nurse will be your care manager, from initial assessment through the course of hospice care. She or he will coordinate your care team of family and friends.

Hospice services generally include:

- Physical Care—Home health care supervised by your hospice nurse that includes medication management to control pain, increase appetite, aid sleep and elevate mood. Hospice provides essential equipment such as a hospital-style bed, commode, urinal or bedpan, mattress pads, dressings—whatever equipment and supplies your diagnosis and condition dictate. Hospice services generally include home health aides to assist with bathing, dressing, and eating. Some hospice services include additional physical comfort therapies such as massage, healing touch, reiki, and reflexology.

- Emotional Support—Hospice social workers, counselors, and volunteers help support you emotionally, helping you with a life review and coming to terms with your approaching death. They also help your family members and friends adjust to losing your presence in this life. Bereavement counseling begins as you approach the end of life. Such counseling continues for your loved ones following your death. Hospice staff also assist in helping you realize your goals during the final months, weeks, and days of your life by assisting you in whatever activity brings you joy and contentment. Music, art, crafts, story-telling, reminiscing, or being present and simply holding hands. Hospice volunteers may also be available for companionship visits and to provide respite for the primary caregiver. Hospice volunteers also may run errands for your caregivers such as picking up groceries. Other hospice volunteers provide pet therapy, bringing their trained and certified pet to your bedside should you desire that type of friendly companionship.

- Spiritual Support—Hospice services include end-of-life counseling by hospice clinical social workers and other therapists to help you and your family prepare and cope with approaching death. Hospice chaplains are available to help address and resolve issues regarding faith, beliefs, and practices of how to face the changes that death brings to the family.

Who Qualifies for Hospice?

You are eligible for hospice care when you have a terminal illness, when treatment is no longer curative, and your life expectancy is considered to be six months or less, assuming the disease takes its normal course. However, when faced with a life-limiting illness, it is best to begin the conversation about hospice right away so you and your loved ones have a good understanding of what hospice offers and you can participate in the planning. Such preplanning can help reduce the stress and strain on all involved as your death approaches.

Paying for Hospice Care

Hospice is paid in full both through the Medicare Hospice Benefit and Medicaid Hospice Benefit. Medicare covered hospice services include equipment such as a hospital bed, bedside commode, walkers or other mobility assistive devices; medications, and home health aides as needed, plus counseling and grief support for the patient and the family. The Veterans Administration also covers hospice services either in full or with minimal co-pay. Many private hospice centers also have policies to accept those who are either under-insured or uninsured.

Free-standing Hospice Centers

Today free-standing hospice inpatient facilities are often designed and decorated to resemble a comfortable home. The beds are often hospital beds, but the rest of the furnishings are very home-like. You can bring pictures and meaningful mementos to decorate your own space in the hospice facility. Some facilities have private rooms, others have shared space. The community hospice facility where I worked had been beautifully converted from a former elementary school. Smaller private rooms were available as well as larger rooms that accommodated up to four people, each of whom had defined space with ceiling-to-floor curtains that could be pulled to surround the bed for additional privacy.

All hospice facilities welcome families and friends. Hospice volunteers help staff provide personal care, help with meals for those unable to feed themselves, and provide entertainment according to individuals' desires. Hospice facilities also often have dogs, cats, or birds so residents who enjoy pets can experience that special type of companionship. Gardens with chairs, benches, or recliners often surround the facility for patients and families to enjoy outdoor visits.

Hospice Respite Care

Hospice "respite care" allows family caregivers to have a brief break. Depending on your insurance, you may receive up to five consecutive days at any one time in an in-patient hospice facility or a skilled nursing home. There may be a small cost-sharing for respite care.

Hospice Care for Children

Unlike adults, children diagnosed with a terminal illness can receive hospice care while they continue to receive curative treatment. While many community hospice services across the country accept children for home care or for inpatient services, currently only a handful of child-specific hospice programs are available. Many families want their child at home, in familiar surroundings, with their parents, siblings, pets and friends. Other families are more comfortable in the familiar surroundings and strong bonds with the staff of the hospital where their child has been treated and want that care to continue. No matter where the terminally ill child is treated, hospice end-of-life care is available. As with adults, advance directives should be in place for a terminally ill child. Community hospice services such as bereavement counseling, support groups for parents and siblings can help navigate the profound grief of the child's death.

Hospice Care for Cancer
People with terminal cancer account for nearly 40% of all hospice patient diagnoses. Hospice care for those with cancer focuses on improving quality of life by controlling symptoms such as pain, fatigue, weakness and body wasting, anxiety, and depression. The majority of cancer patients admitted to hospice require pain control that can be achieved within the first 48 hours following admission. Comfort care often includes gentle skin care as well as medications to help stimulate your appetite and mood, if wanted.

Hospice Care for Heart Disease
Hospice care for those with heart disease focuses on improving quality of life by controlling pain, shortness

of breath, nausea, fatigue, swelling, weight gain, anxiety, and depression. Hospice nurses have specialized pulmonary training to help the person control their symptoms in the home including cough, congestion, constipation, shortness of breath, and swelling. In-home respiratory medications are provided to help control symptoms; the same medications as those used in emergency rooms such as inhalers, morphine, and supplemental oxygen.

Hospice Care for Alzheimer's Disease or Dementia

We have no cure for Alzheimer's disease and other forms of dementia, therefore, people with any form of dementia qualify for hospice care. Generally forms of dementia progress slowly but relentlessly. From the mild forgetfulness of normal aging, people with true dementia progress through recognizable stages. Neurologists use various assessments to make the probable diagnosis of Alzheimer's or other dementia. However, the diagnosis of Alzheimer's dementia is only definitively confirmed following the person's death through an autopsy.

Graduating from Hospice

If the disease seems to be in remission and your condition improves over the first six months of hospice care, you can be discharged from hospice. You can choose to return to aggressive therapy or simply go about your daily life until you need to return to hospice care. Medicare and most private insurance will allow additional coverage for this purpose. Should you wish to remain in hospice care, your hospice physician and your primary physician will recertify your eligibility for hospice based on your continued life-limiting illness. Under Medicare, you are certified for two ninety-day periods, followed by an unlimited number of sixty day periods.

In 2006, the famed humorist, Art Buchwald, epitomized hospice care benefits. In his book, *Too Soon to Say Goodbye*, Art recounted that by 80 years of age, part of a leg had been amputated, his kidneys had completely failed, and his doctors prescribed dialysis, a procedure he would have to endure several times a week for the remainder of his life. Art refused. He had a totally different idea of what made his life meaningful and extended treatment did not fit in that picture. Instead, Art was discharged from ICU and admitted to a Washington, D.C. hospice facility where he proceeded to "have the time of his life." He improved so much that he was discharged from hospice after a five-month stay. He returned to his home to "resume the life of a funny old man" and to finish his book with the intent of "making hospice a household word." He did complete his book and many months later returned to hospice for a brief stay before he finally succumbed to kidney failure.

All Hospices are Not the Same

As with hospitals and nursing homes, certified hospices are required by private insurance companies, Medicare,

Medicaid, and the Veterans Administration to provide a basic level of care. However, the amount and quality of services may vary significantly from one hospice to another. To find the best hospice for your needs, ask your doctor, other healthcare professionals, social workers, clergy, or friends who have received care for a family member. The National Hospice and Palliative Care Organization has a search feature to help you locate a hospice by city or zip code and hospice facility name.

Consumer Reports suggests using the following criteria when considering hospice services:

- Medicare approval
- Not-for-profit status
- 20 or more years of experience.
- Hospice-certified nurses and doctors on staff and available 24 hours per day
- Palliative-care consultants who can begin care if you're not yet ready for hospice
- An inpatient unit, where patients can go if symptoms can't be managed at home
- Ability to provide care in nursing homes and assisted living residences

If you have done that type of homework and find yourself dissatisfied with a chosen hospice service, make sure you communicate your expectations and desires to the hospice team. It is important to trust that your nurse and the team will be responsive, especially as death draws near. Make sure you are comfortable with the communication and feel confident in the services. If the hospice you have chosen does not or cannot satisfy your needs and desires, do not hesitate to choose another hospice service.

If you love me, why would you leave me
when you can stay a little longer?

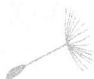

CHAPTER 6

PHYSICIAN-ASSISTED DEATH (PAD)

One of the choices now more readily available in our modern world is Physician-Assisted Death (PAD). Do you recall the drama surrounding Dr. Jack Kevorkian, who famously publicly championed a terminal patient's right to die by physician-assisted suicide? He was arrested in 1998 for his part in the voluntary euthanasia of a man (reportedly there were many) and sentenced to jail for second-degree murder. Kevorkian served eight years of a 10-25 year prison sentence.

My, how times have changed.

Kevorkian believed physicians are responsible for alleviating the suffering of patients, and on that much I will agree with him. But I am not a strong proponent for the physician-assisted death he advocated.

With great interest, in 2014 I followed the end-of-life saga of Brittany Maynard, a 29-year-old who suffered unremitting seizures caused by her glioblastoma, a type of brain tumor for which we have no cure. Maynard, an advocate for the legalization of assisted death, made the decision to have physician-assisted death in order to control the process and timing of her death. She had to move from California to Oregon, because Oregon was one of only five states where such means was authorized at the time. She wanted to receive a prescription from a physician for medication that she could self-ingest to end her dying process. This process was dubbed "death with dignity." Please hear my clarion call now: There are MANY ways to "die with dignity!" I am a fierce advocate for hospice, the core philosophy being dignity and peace and choice.

While I understood why Brittany so strongly advocated for her own physician-assisted death, my heart ached for her and her family that they did not experience the compassionate comfort care that hospice provides the dying and those they love.

Hospice care does not hasten death but relieves the physical, emotional, and spiritual suffering that is part of terminal illness. Ideally, hospice care addresses all aspects of suffering and improves quality of life right up to the last breath. If I am diagnosed with a terminal illness, I know I will choose to receive the comfort care that hospice provides. However, I have watched with dismay through recent years as more and more states pass legislation approving physician-assisted death (PAD). I understand that we, as independent adults, want to control every aspect of our lives including our death. We don't want to feel pain nor do we want to linger, being a burden to anyone. But having a physician assist us in ending our life in order to end our suffering is the direct opposite of the multi-dimensional comfort care that hospice service offers us. Our pain can always be relieved. Our friends and family can gather to provide physical and emotional support to us, and each other, while they prepare themselves for losing us.

Physical pain is just one aspect of suffering we fear when we contemplate the end of our life. There are many other aspects of our final illness that we dread. Having enjoyed being strong and independent, we fight against losing control of our strength and abilities. Having a terminal illness changes our sense of self. We would rather care for others than have them care for us. We fear the loss of dignity as our physical body weakens. As parents and grandparents, we have bathed our babies and wiped their bottoms, but it is hard to adjust to receiving such care from our adult children and grandchildren. We do not want to be a burden for our loved ones but our final illness often requires us to have help with toileting, bathing, and even eating. Faced with the specter of suffering that terminal illness may bring, some of us may contemplate ending our lives by suicide rather than a natural death.

This breaks my heart.

I cherish the memories I have of caring for each of my parents in their final illnesses. Bed baths with foot soaks and massages became a prayerful time. Being able to do "hands on" care while playing their favorite instrumental music helped ease my sorrow because I could actively help them. I knew it would not be long before I would not have the opportunity to do those things for them ever again. Speaking softly while cleaning and caressing their fragile skin allowed me to say the important things that were in my heart. I was able to say the essential messages Dr. Byock suggests we say as death approaches; "I love you" and "I know you love me;" "I am sorry for the pain I caused you and I forgive you for the pain you caused me." "I will keep you and your love in my heart always and look forward to when we meet again." Had my parents chosen physician-assisted death, I would have missed all those moments I still cherish decades later.

The legalities of physician-assisted death especially concerns me for those with a life-limiting illness who cannot speak for themselves such as those with mental or profound emotional challenges. Rather than legislating death, I hope those of us in the "Baby Boomer" generation, and younger generations, put much more emphasis on preserving our lives to our natural end through education in palliative care and hospice services so we dispel all of our end-of-life fears.

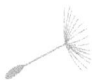

Death is not to be feared.
Death is to be faced, with dignity, and deep
abiding love for all involved.

Hospice is a philosophy of care that values Life from the moment it begins to the moment it ends.
Dame Cicely Saunders

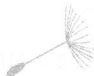

CHAPTER 7

A HOSPICE HANDBOOK

Making the decision to forego aggressive or curative treatment and have hospice care while you still have strength and energy gives you the opportunity to continue to do beloved activities at home that you would not necessarily be able to do in a hospital setting.

In the *Journal of Clinical Oncology*, Dr. Rahul Bannerjee writes about a patient whose lymphoma did not respond to any of the many aggressive treatments the medical team had tried. They did not have any other treatment to offer her and recommended hospice. The patient asked if she would be able to tend the plants in her garden and make meals from her home-grown vegetables. The medical team assured her the hospice team would help control her pain and nausea so her dream would be feasible. Finally, the patient chose hospice care.

But all the aggressive treatments had left her tremendously fatigued. The hospice team was able to control her pain and nausea, but her profound weakness depleted her of the energy she needed to even visit her garden by wheelchair, much less actually tend plants or prepare a meal. Both she and her medical team had waited too long to consider hospice when she still had the strength to accomplish her end of life goals.

The right time for considering hospice is different for every person but the NHPCO suggests engaging hospice services when you:

- Have frequent ER visits or hospitalizations due to chronic, life-limiting illness.
- Want to transition from acute care to end of life care.
- Want to be cared for at home or in a home-like setting rather than a hospital.
- Have questions about or need help with your own pain management and medications.
- Have a diminished quality of life due to illness or the effects of treatment.

If you are mulling over any of those questions, it is time to call hospice services to start the conversation. Also if your caregiver is exhausted from being the primary party responsible for your at-home care, it's time to talk to hospice. Remember, you qualify to receive hospice services at no cost through Medicare, Medicaid, or your private supplemental insurance when your physician expects you will die within six months. Since it is often difficult for doctors to predict when death may occur, especially in older adults with multiple chronic illnesses that cannot be cured, hospice provides comfort care that many times extends life beyond the original prediction. If that happens, your doctor will recertify you as qualifying for services for as long as you need such care until your death.

Choosing a Hospice

Choosing the right hospice service is similar to choosing your doctor. Perhaps the best way is by word-of-mouth, particularly if a family member or trusted friend recommends one because of their experience with that hospice provider. Your doctor may have a preferred choice or have a list of local hospices. If you are already hospitalized, the hospital discharge planner or social worker will provide a list of local hospice agencies.

Make an informational appointment with the one(s) that appeal to you. These questions can help you determine which hospice service is right for you:

1. How quickly is a care plan developed and put into place?

2. How quickly can pain and/or symptoms be relieved or managed?

3. How quickly will the hospice respond if pain or other symptoms are not adequately relieved?

4. What is expected of the family caregiver; will hospice provide caregiver training?

5. Are there services, medications, or equipment that the family needs to provide?

6. Are there out-of-pocket expenses the family should anticipate?

7. Are medications delivered to the home or does the family have to pick them up at a pharmacy?

8. How often will the hospice team member visit and for how long?

9. Is inpatient care available outside of the home?

10. Who to contact at hospice about any aspect of care?

11. What hospice services are provided, including bereavement support?

12. Is quality of care measured; can the hospice share the quality data?

Assessment

You, your spouse/family member, or your doctor can make the initial inquiry to hospice. If you or your loved one makes the initial contact, the hospice team will reach out to your doctor to confirm that hospice care is appropriate.

A hospice case worker, often a nurse or social worker, will visit you in your home or wherever you reside to begin the qualifying paperwork. A consent for service form must be signed as well as insurance forms, similar to forms required when being admitted to a hospital. The case worker will explain the admitting process, assess your physical needs and review medications. She or he will recommend any additional equipment, such as a hospital bed, bedside commode, and other assistive devices and help make arrangements to obtain the necessary equipment for you. Depending on when you begin hospice services, your need for equipment may be minimal at first and gradually increase as illness progresses. The aim is to provide you with everything you will need to live in a safe, clean, home environment until death, or until you decide to move to a hospice facility or hospital-based hospice care unit if that becomes your choice.

You and your family will be supported by a hospice and palliative care certified nurse who will manage your care, schedule hospice aides to provide personal care as needed, as well as coordinate hospice volunteers to visit. Your hospice nurse will develop a care plan customized to your needs and desires, including the number of family and friend caregivers involved and the amount of caregiving required. The care plan also helps the hospice team know how much hospice-provided support will be needed. Depending on when hospice care begins, it may not be necessary for someone to be with you at all times.

As your illness advances, the hospice team will usually recommend that someone always be home and available to you. Typically a family member provides most of your care at home. However, hospice service also includes home health aides to help with personal care and volunteers who can run errands and provide primary family caregivers a break. Hospice staff is on call for emergencies or concerns 24/7, 365 days a year. If you require more care than can be provided in the home, hospice care in a free-standing facility or skilled nursing home is often an option. Some acute care hospitals also have a palliative care hospice care patient unit where traditional hospice services of comfort care for the dying are provided.

Pain Management

Pain management is the hallmark of hospice comfort care. Your hospice physician and nurse will make sure you are comfortable. As Dr. Byock says, "Physical pain can always be controlled." Pain medication such as morphine can be given in much higher doses without the risks and side effects experienced by a person without terminal illness.

Some medications may limit your ability to carry on conversations. If your goal is to be alert, your hospice physician and nurse will revise the medication plan to control your pain and still allow you to converse. Sometimes, the illness itself can cause such intense pain that the only way to relieve it is to induce unconsciousness or a "medical coma." Your hospice physician and nurse will consult with you and your loved ones if such a measure is needed to make you comfortable.

Physical comfort is only one aspect of hospice care. Your emotional and spiritual comfort is also of paramount importance. Because hospice is focused on providing you with the highest quality of life possible, the staff will want to know as much as possible about your favorite things—from your favorite foods, pets, and friends, to helping you with favorite activities and routines you most enjoy so you can continue to enjoy them for as long as possible.

Signs of Approaching Death

One of the deepest fears for family and friends caring for someone in home hospice care is knowing when death is imminent. Understanding what to expect helps allay those fears.

As in every aspect of life, the dying process encompasses our physical and emotional selves. Often the emotional signs of approaching death precede the physical signs of the body shutting down. Your hospice team will coach you and your family and friends regarding these emotional and physical signs.

Generally in a terminal illness, the active dying process begins one to three months prior to the actual death. Both emotional and physical signs become more pronounced one to three weeks before the patient dies.

Emotional Signs of Approaching Death

The dying patient may:

- Engage in a life review, retelling cherished memories of childhood or earlier adulthood.
- See and speak to relatives or friends who have preceded them in death.
- Offer beloved personal belongings to family members and friends, to experience the joy and gratitude such gifts generate rather than have those items just listed in their will.
- Become increasingly less social, declining visits from friends and neighbors even if they have welcomed such visits earlier in their illness.
- Withdraw from immediate surroundings; may refuse personal care or become more difficult to care for.

Physical Signs of Approaching Death

The person may be nearing death when they:

- Become increasingly less active
- Eat and drink less
- Void and defecate less
- Talk less
- Sleep more
- Become weaker
- Become colder to the touch, their skin will become pale and sometimes mottled with blue and purple patches

- Become confused, speak incoherently or become delirious
- Thrash around in bed, shifting from side to side
- Have a change in breathing pattern; either faster or slower breathing, may gasp for air or have gradually longer pauses between breaths

These emotional and physical signs are common, normal, and expected. In the natural world, animals usually withdraw from their pack, pride, herd, or flock. They are less active, and cease eating and drinking well before they take their final breath. As the signs of approaching death become apparent, your hospice nurse will be available to help comfort and soothe you and your family and provide comfort measures that address both emotional and physical needs.

Comfort Care for the Dying

Comfort care measures that family, friends and hospice provide to meet the dying person's emotional needs include:

- Encouraging the dying person to discuss their life by asking questions or simply listening and acknowledging a well-lived life.
- Acknowledging how comforting it is to be present to see them and hear their voice.
- Graciously accepting the gift or heirloom and saying how much having such a gift means.

- Limiting bedside visits to only those few family or friends who are essential for care near the end of life.
- Providing only necessary personal care without causing undue distress.
- Playing favorite music, with soft lighting and desired bedding to maximize comfort.

Comfort care that addresses the physical signs of approaching death includes:

- As appetite and thirst wane, there is no need to force food or fluids; lips and mouth are kept moist using a wet washcloth and lip balm, mouth swabs.
- Keep bed linen clean and dry to protect the skin, use bed pads to wick moisture away from perineum and buttocks.
- The typical hospice "medication comfort kit" commonly includes drugs, often:
  - Haldol (halopurinol) to relieve restlessness, agitation, or thrashing.
  - Atropine drops or Levsin (hyoscyamine sulfate) to relieve rapid or noisy breathing (commonly called a "death rattle").
  - Morphine sulfate to relieve pain and ease rapid/gasping breathing or panting.
  - Compazine (prochlorperazine) or Phenergan (promethazine) to relieve nausea.

I have never wanted to administer a soothing drug more than during the final weekend of my dad's life. The hospice case manager was scheduled to assess him for admittance to hospice service on Monday but my dad began thrashing in his sleep on Saturday night. He appeared to be asleep but could not stop moving, throwing himself from side to side. My heart ached for the lack of the medicine I knew would help him and his restlessness. We had waited far too long to initiate hospice care for the father I deeply loved. As a nurse steeped in knowledge of elder care and hospice, I felt I had terribly failed my father at the most crucial time. My purpose in writing this book is to help ensure that no other daughter, son, brother, sister or spouse feels that sense of guilt or regret.

I am forever grateful that years later, my father-in-law's death epitomized what hospice comfort care provides. Walter was hospitalized at age 93 with end-stage heart disease and his physicians had nothing more to offer him. His wife, June, knew she did not have the physical strength or emotional stamina to care for him at home. She also knew the local hospice agency had a beautiful in-patient facility close to their home. The case manager assessed Walter while he was still hospitalized and arranged for him to have non-emergency medical transport to the facility at discharge. The hospice nursing staff were very attentive, addressing every physical and emotional need for both Walter and June.

The family gathered from near and far to say farewell. All of his children, their spouses, and grandchildren arrived at his bedside. Walter was in and out of consciousness. We all shared favorite memories of family times together with him. We talked and laughed about the fun we all had together through the years. His nurses checked on him, repositioning him when he seemed restless and quickly provided medication to ease his breathing when needed. June asked my husband and his sister to accompany her to the funeral home to finalize plans. Neither sibling wanted to leave their dad so close to death but they both knew she needed their support. We are all certain that my father-in-law knew his wife needed that support more than he did at that time. So the threesome left while several other family members and I remained at his bedside. Walter had just been turned onto his left side and I was sitting by the head of his bed. Knowing he could still hear me, I softly whispered a favorite joke we had shared in the past. I will always remember his soft, single chuckle before he drew his final breath. I am comforted, as was his wife and the entire family, knowing Walter died laughing, in comfort and in peace.

When Death Comes

The admitting coordinator or hospice nurse gives instructions regarding who to contact if death is near or when death occurs. It is important to remember that there is no need to contact emergency medical services (EMS), the police, or any other service when a patient receiving hospice care dies. Death in hospice is not an emergency. It is a carefully planned and anticipated event. Your hospice nurse or a member of the hospice team will contact the physician and if directed, the funeral home. Hospice services will remove any and all equipment provided and remaining medications. Your hospice team will shift focus from providing patient end-of-life care to providing grief and bereavement support for you and your family for however long such support is needed.

I once saw an acronym for Hospice—Helping Others Slip Into Calm Eternity—and it resonated with me. The goal of my work, and this book, is to allow people to gracefully exit this life and enter calm eternity. I have witnessed many peaceful deaths in hospice care and I am on a mission to spread the word that this type of peaceful passing is available.

There is another quote from an unknown source that I like: "Healing does not mean that a cure will occur but that the heart will come to rest." When it comes to matters of the heart, nothing is more stirring than death. From all my years as a nurse, I know it is possible to achieve a death with pain under control, with faculties still present, with one's desires being fulfilled.

The choice is always yours, but do know you have a choice. You do not have to die in a sterile environment surrounded by strangers. You can go home to be with those you love, and who love you. You can eat, drink, and live on your terms, until you are no longer living. You can create a death that helps your family and friends ease into life without you because they know you were satisfied with your final days. For all the advances in modern medicine, nothing can keep us alive forever, but we do have the ability to plan and prepare for death. That is an opportunity we should take full advantage of.

When we are no longer able to change a situation,
we are challenged to change ourselves.
Victor E. Frankl

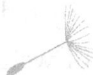

CHAPTER 8

RESILIENCE IN GRIEF

Hal began experiencing ever-increasing fatigue which he chalked up to normal aging since he had recently turned seventy. However, on a weekend car trip to New York City with his wife, Helen, his fatigue became overwhelming. Hal could not enjoy the city tours he had planned or the restaurants' fine foods. He slept the entire trip home while Helen drove, deeply worried about her husband. Upon returning home and going to the hospital, Hal and Helen were stunned when the ER doctor immediately hospitalized him and told him his diagnosis—acute myeloid leukemia (AML).

True to his courageous fighting spirit, Hal explored treatment options and agreed with his oncologist's recommendation for an aggressive course of chemotherapy and a stem cell transplant. At his age, Hal really needed a perfect match to achieve complete remission, and although his son was not a perfect match, Hal and his medical team and the family agreed to go ahead.

The harsh chemotherapy reduced his immune system to zero and he lost a lot of weight very quickly, but Hal and his family celebrated the day his son's stem cells were transfused. They all believed that the worst was over. But despite his medical remission, Hal suffered debilitating treatment side effects unrelieved by the many medications prescribed. After being discharged home, Hal had to return to the outpatient department for blood draws three times per week, trips that left him profoundly wiped out. As the months unfolded, he slowly managed to regain some strength and stamina, yet Hal had little true quality of life.

Lab tests soon revealed the AML had relapsed. The prognosis for patients with relapsed AML ranges, but with Hal being in his seventies achieving a second remission was extremely unlikely. Instead of having a frank discussion of these sobering statistics, Hal's physicians told him about two new targeted therapy drugs recently approved by the FDA. Always a fighter, Hal opted to try the new therapy. For his remaining months, Hal and Helen both endured greater suffering as he valiantly fought his illness and new treatment side effects. Though he finally did make decisions about his funeral and burial, Hal did not agree to stop acute care treatment in favor of comfort care. Their daughter broached the subject of hospice as she witnessed her dad's steady decline but Hal would not consider it, nor did his medical team ever suggest stopping treatment. As Hal grew ever weaker, the signs of worsening AML were apparent. He spent most of his days sleeping when he returned home from his many appointments. One day Hal finally admitted to Helen that he was simply waiting to die. But even then, neither Hal nor his medical team discussed hospice.

On Christmas morning, Hal was too weak to move out of his recliner. His family gathered in the living room as he slept. Hal awakened and seemed to enjoy the quiet festivities. Then suddenly his arm started jerking, contracting with movements he could not control. He said he was not in pain but he simply could not control his arm. Frightened by his new symptom, Helen called 911 and Hal was transported to the ER. Helen wisely gave a copy of Hal's living will to the ambulance crew. Though Hal had not considered hospice, he had decided not to be resuscitated if his heart or breathing ceased. Helen declined the ER doctor's suggestion that Hal undergo a CT scan. Hal was moved to a private room on the oncology unit where Helen stayed with Hal through the night. During the next day, the family began to talk about hospice care but by evening, Hal was unconscious. Hal died the next morning.

We all suffer, the patient and the family, and we all have resilience we may not be aware of. Helen, a strong woman, had championed her husband's chosen course of treatment even though she would have made other choices had she been faced with an incurable illness. And despite knowing in her heart that Hal's death was near, she was shocked and heartbroken when he died.

Resilience is a dynamic process of adapting well in the face of adversity, trauma, and tragedy. Hal showed great physical and emotional resilience in the face of a devastating illness. He suffered physically but his will remained strong. Even when wheelchair-bound during his outpatient visits for transfusions, he mustered energy to visit other patients and families who had become friends during the many months of his treatment. Helen showed immense resilience as Hal's devoted caregiver throughout the course of his illness.

Helen was deeply bereft after Hal's death. She had enjoyed a 51-year marriage with him. Before she could even think of building a new life on her own, Helen had to take time to grieve.

Harvard professor, J. William Worden, counsels that the death of someone close to us is something that is not gotten "over." The work of grief involves learning to live with and adjust to the loss. Grieving is a whole body-mind experience and takes physical, emotional, and spiritual effort. Redefining and recreating a purposeful, meaningful life poses enormous physical, social, psychological, and spiritual challenges. According to Worden, there may be a sense that we are never finished with grief, but by working toward realistic goals, we can eventually feel hopeful again and rekindle our interest in living our life. This of course takes time, and there is no set deadline. To see grief as tremendously hard work actually can make it easier to face.

Dr. Worden uses the term "tasks" of grieving and they include:

1. accept the reality of the loss;
2. work through the pain of grief;
3. adjust to an environment in which the deceased is missing;
4. emotionally "relocate" the deceased.

He explains "emotionally relocating" our dead loved one is an ongoing process that continues throughout our life. While their physical presence is gone from our life, they remain forever with us. Death does not end our relationship, and love endures beyond death, but the work of moving through our grief requires our commitment and active participation.

Survivorship suffering is often complicated by feelings of guilt and regret. By planning for your death and making your wishes known, you can eliminate the "if only" or "what if" scenarios that grieving loved ones ponder. When you die, you do not want your beloveds to be riddled with guilt and regret. The "woulda, shoulda, coulda" thoughts can be put to rest when your family knows that they carried out your wishes.

None of us wants to be haunted by thoughts of what we would have done had we only known that death would come that soon. Hence the need for Advanced Directives. The term may sound sterile, but they are instead a love letter.

Taking time to grieve and cope with the consequences of loss helps us begin to reconcile our suffering. From that suffering we build and bolster our resilience. Resilience is a continual learning process of adapting in the midst of and in response to Life's adversities.

Helen slowly adjusted to her new life without Hal. Early in her bereavement, her children and grandchildren kept close company with Helen. Gradually, she began to reweave her new life into the tapestry she and Hal had created a half a century ago. She started by rescuing two dogs from a local shelter. Walking them daily in the neighborhood not only provided needed physical exercise but also the camaraderie of neighbors and friends. Helen took trips to see siblings and life-long friends. With each trip, she grew stronger in her independence, and in enjoyment of her accomplishments.

As Elizabeth Kübler-Ross and David Kessler wrote, "You will not "get over" the loss of a loved one; you will learn to live with it. You will heal and you will build yourself around the loss you have suffered. You will be whole again but you will never be the same. Nor should you be the same nor would you want to."

Resilience is our ability to adjust to life's changes and challenges. Unlike a rubber band that returns to its previous shape after being stretched, our hearts and minds do not "bounce back" from the grief we encounter as we age. As we experience our own physical losses in aging, facing a terminal illness, or the deaths of others, we do not recover but we adjust. We develop a "new normal" life after the loss of a loved one. Our lives are forever changed but the acute gut-wrenching pain slowly lessens as we continue to adjust. Time helps the gaping wound in our heart and spirit to close.

Post-Traumatic Growth

As we get stronger, we can achieve what scientists and counselors call post-traumatic growth. Post-traumatic growth goes beyond resilience into positive personal change. As Helen continued to move through her widowhood, she not only demonstrated resilience of mind and body, but also post-traumatic growth by continuing to pursue her own life-long dreams and being open to forming new relationships.

Like post-traumatic stress, post-traumatic growth is not universal, there are various ways to grow. Researchers at the National Cancer Institute (NCI) are studying the positive life changes that occur through the traumatic and life-changing experience of cancer. Their studies show that people experience different types of growth, including:

- Improved relations with others. Living with a life-threatening illness such as cancer may deepen connection with family or friends. It may also be easier to connect with others who have had a similar traumatic event.

- New life experiences. Living with cancer may change previous priorities, resulting in different life choices, such as a career change or overcoming a fear.

- A greater appreciation for life. Living with cancer may provide a deeper value of life itself, a deeper appreciation of the world, or result in a new feeling of vulnerability to death. This awareness may renew or increase appreciation of being in this world.

- A sense of personal strength. Living with cancer may result in the development of more mental strength and a feeling of empowerment in triumphing over suffering.

- Spiritual development. Living with cancer may result in a greater interest in religion or increasing a spiritual depth to life.

All of these factors can be applied to the post-traumatic growth of grief. Instead of saying "living with cancer," replace that phrase with "living with loss" and apply it to those five growth factors above.

As much as it sounds trite, or even cruel, life does go on. Grief can bring spiritual development, a sense of personal strength, a greater appreciation for life, new life experiences, and improved relationships with others. There are countless ways to work through your grief. You do it in your way, in your time. The very fact that you get out of bed day after day is a sign of resilience. In time, you are open to new possibilities.

Helen found a deep and abiding friendship with a former high school friend, Dave, who is a widower. As their friendship rekindled, they felt a deep spiritual connection, having grown up in the same city, with mutual friends and similar experiences, and both supporting and comforting their spouses through their final illnesses. Now both Helen and Dave are growing beyond their traumatic bereavement experiences. Each are more accepting of the changes that have been wrought in their lives. Both are feeling stronger physically and emotionally and are beginning to embrace what Life still has in store for them. While still lovingly honoring their spouses, both Helen and Dave are beginning to grow and thrive in their new lives.

How do we triumph over suffering and increase our resilience?

NCI's research in post-traumatic growth suggests the following ways to promote your own resilience and experience positive personal growth following traumatic experiences such as deep bereavement:

Reduce your anxiety and tension caused by the traumatic grief

- Use relaxation techniques—meditation, massage, deep breathing techniques
- Get regular physical exercise you enjoy
- Maintain a healthy diet to nourish your body as you heal your heart and spirit
- Talk honestly with supportive family and friends about your feelings
- Focus on the present rather than dwelling on past regrets

Restore your sense of safety

- A trusted counselor, social worker, chaplain, or spiritual advisor can help assuage your fears and help you realize that while life may be changed, life is still very much worth living

Connect with others

- Consider joining a support group of people who understand the shared experience. Hospice services include grief counseling on a one-on-one basis as well as groups, for widows and widowers, and for those who mourn the death of a parent, siblings, or child.

- Support groups are available for cancer and most other illnesses and conditions, as well as groups for other physical, emotional or spiritual health concerns and meet either in-person or online.

Create a resilient life vision

- Think about what you have learned from your traumatic grief experience.
- Make concrete plans about how you will live more fully, pursuing your own dreams.

Building resiliency and strength, whether physical or emotional takes time. Five sit-ups does not result in a sculpted "six-pack" abdomen any more than walking a block prepares you to run a marathon. Attempting new skills such as meditation and relaxation takes effort. But each of those activities are a beginning point. As John Denver sang years ago, "Some days are diamonds, some days are stone." But as the days go by, your spirit grows more resilient as you work to accept and adjust to the "new normal" life you are creating. There is no standard timeline. You will live and grow into your new resilience your own way. One step at a time, one day at a time, until you have a moment when you see the strength and resilience you once thought was impossible. As St.

Francis of Assisi said, "Start by doing what's necessary; then do what's possible, and suddenly you are doing the impossible."

You gave me a forever within the numbered days.
John Green

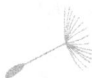

CHAPTER 9

CELEBRATION OF LIFE

Often grief and bereavement is still raw and consuming at the time of the funeral or memorial service. Even when death is anticipated and the dying person participated in advance planning of their own funeral, grief can be overwhelming during the final services because it signals saying "goodbye." But we do not actually ever say a final farewell. Our beloved never truly leaves us. Recalling our happy (and the not-always-so-happy) times is a source of comfort as we begin to navigate our life without their physical presence. As the author Mitch Albom says, "Life has to end, Love doesn't."

To honor our love, we often need a public celebration of the life of our deceased. And sometimes the dying person truly wants to be a real part of it. A relatively new end-of-life trend has emerged in the past few years. Some folks who have accepted that their illness is terminal plan a celebration of life prior to their death so they can be part of their own "memorial" service. The dying person gathers family and friends to rejoice in their shared love, tell stories and reminisce while they are still able to enjoy the party. While death is never an easy experience, being able to celebrate together is not only comforting to the one who is facing imminent death, but family and friends are later consoled in their bereavement by the photos taken and memories made during this celebration.

With my experience as a "caring clown" and involvement in the Association for Applied and Therapeutic Humor (AATH), I expect to plan a fun and funny celebration of my life when my death nears. I will have red sponge clown noses for family and friends to wear as they share silly stories of our times together, hilarious memories of my Lucy Ricardo tendencies, tell me cornball jokes and puns, and sing songs off key. The soundtrack of my life will liven the party with favorite music from Beethoven and Bach to Jimmy Buffett, from the Rat Pack to Vivaldi and every genre in between. I expect there will be tears but also lots of laughter. Like the line from "Steel Magnolias," laughter through tears is my favorite emotion. The smiling faces of those I hold most dear will be my celebration as I transition to eternity.

My husband has a totally different vision for the end of his life. He does not want "the gathering of the clan" to mourn at a formal funeral service. Neither does he wish to have a celebration of life party prior to his death. Instead, he would like his family and friends, wherever they are, to simply raise a glass of their favorite beverage and think of a time when he and they were together, enjoying each other's company.

Traditional funeral services in a place of worship or funeral home or internment site are generally somber occasions, but such services may be comforting for survivors who appreciate the sanctity of tradition. Some people choose to hold the service shortly after the death of their loved one and then plan a celebration of life weeks, or months, after the funeral. Some opt for a celebration of life instead of a traditional funeral service at all. And for some, spending time at the gravesite or columbarium can bring peace and comfort.

There are endless ways to honor and grieve and celebrate. Having an evening candle-lighting ceremony can set a soothing mood. Making a "memory jar" by having family and friends write a favorite memory creates a gift that will continue to bring comfort for years to come. Continued celebrations of life can be on a birthday, wedding anniversary, anniversary of death, or other significant times. The location can be anywhere that is special to our loved one and to us.

Ways to honor a person are as varied as individual passions and interests. You can plant a tree or a garden of favorite flowers and plants. Or give family and friends seed packets of favorite flowers or vegetables to plant in their own yard in the loved one's memory. You can create a playlist of their favorite songs to share with others or to simply listen to yourself to soothe your heart and feel closer to them. Make a memory box of pictures of that person or photos taken by them. Get together with friends and family to make a favorite menu and share a special meal; reminisce about feasts from the past; go to a favorite restaurant to enjoy a meal together, reminiscing about previous get-togethers there. Make a quilt from fabric squares from their t-shirts, ties, or clothing. Watch their favorite movies or funny shows. Distribute humorous items that made our loved one laugh. There are endless ways to celebrate the love and special moments. Some set up scholarships. Others plan an annual event supporting a favorite charity. There are countless opportunities to continue to celebrate the life of those we love throughout our remaining years.

Michael had cancer for a few years before he died. He stated he did not want any kind of funeral or memorial service. His wife, Ruth, honored all his wishes on how he wanted to die and he had a peaceful death at home. After a month, Ruth realized she needed to have a celebration of life service. She went to his grave and told him, "This is not for you, it's for me." She knew he would understand. Ruth rented a hall and had friends sing his favorite songs, read his favorite poems, and they all toasted to his wonderful life and how much they loved him. Ruth was able to work though her grieving process better by holding a celebration of the man she loved so deeply.

Perhaps you want to be cremated and have your ashes scattered across your fishing pond. Maybe you want Scottish bagpipes played at your funeral. You might want your family and friends to dance a conga line at your celebration life party. Make your wishes known.

Many people now take part in the planning of their own funerals, celebrations, and even write their own obituaries. This exercise can be a lovely way to review your life and share cherished memories with friends and family, and make this task one less thing that your survivors have to face upon your death.

With acceptance, anticipation, and compassionate planning, you can experience a peaceful death and give that peace to those who surround you with love. A serene death with no regrets does not happen on its own. You must face the normal end-of-life process and decide in advance what care you want when you face your final illness.

The greatest gift you can give yourself and those you love is to recognize that you are mortal and will die. Do the advance planning and preparation necessary for a loving and thoughtful end to the life you have lived and loved.

No regrets, in life and in death, that is Love's last act. Do this for you. Do this for those you love. As Thomas Campbell said, "To live in hearts we leave behind is not to die."

Love lives on. Show family and friends your love. Plan for your death.

They will forever thank you.

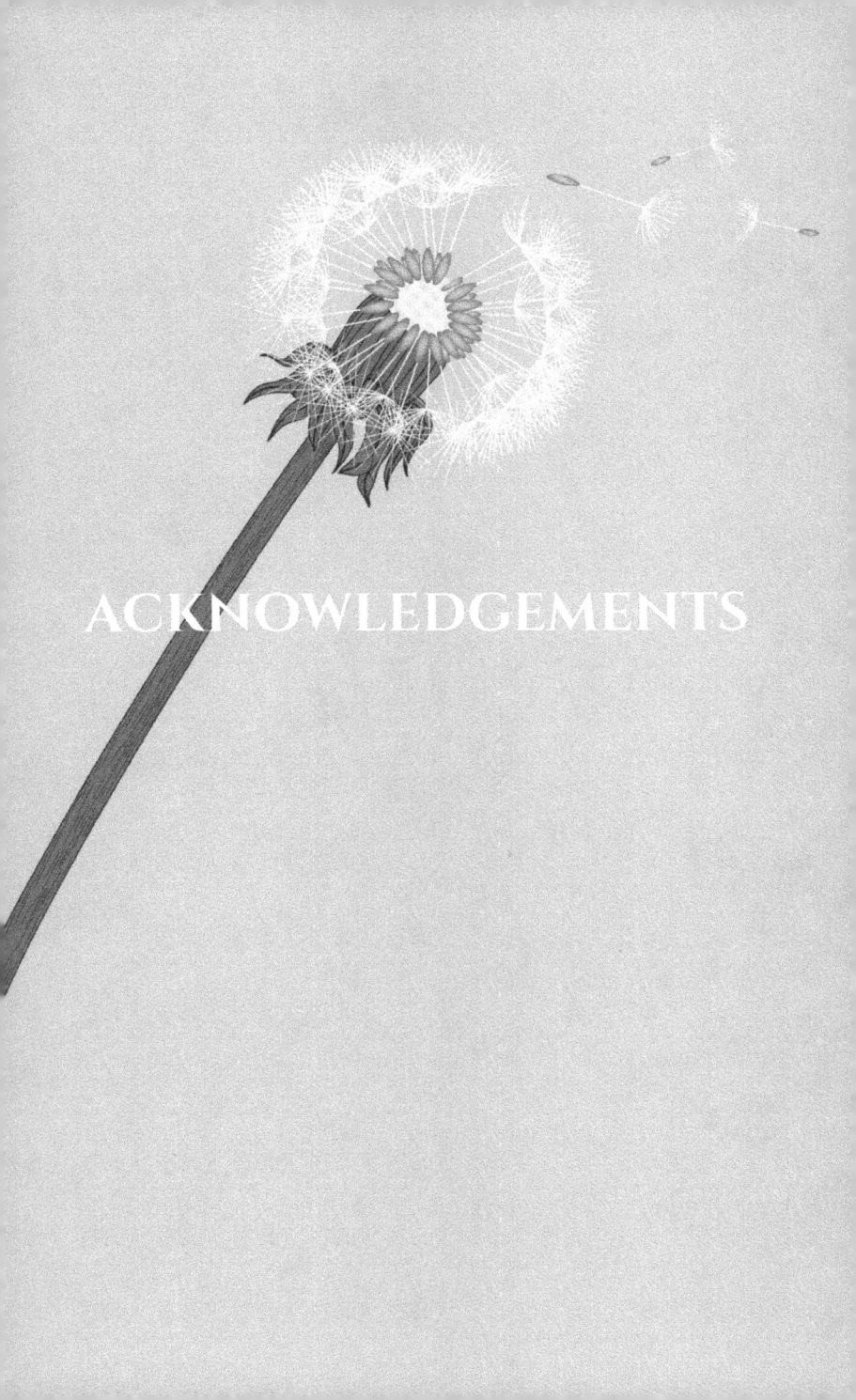

ACKNOWLEDGEMENTS

ACKNOWLEDGEMENTS

I must begin by thanking my dear friend and fellow nurse, Cheryl Fell (also known as Nurse FUNShine), who I know through the Association for Applied and Therapeutic Humor (AATH). As nurses, health educators, and "caring clowns," Cheryl and I are both committed to helping people thrive at every age and also have a peaceful death. I confided in her I had been contemplating writing about end of life care. She gave me the encouragement and needed nudge to get started writing. Had Cheryl not motivated me to document my fervent desire for people to contemplate, plan, and experience a serene death, this book would not have been written. Thank you, Cheryl! I can never say it enough! Thank you!

I also thank Kelly Simmons, a champion encourager as well as extraordinary editor. Her belief in my ability to write this book made me believe it too. From my scattered ideas and patients' stories, Kelly created a cohesive book that fully expresses my passion for ensuring a peaceful death. Lisa DeSpain's cover artistry perfectly illustrates the natural cycle of life with the dandelion being a symbol of emotional healing and peace.

I am profoundly grateful to Carol O'Toole whose insistence on including complementary therapies of massage and meditation in her breast cancer treatment care plan forever changed the way I cared for patients.

I am indebted to the patients and families I met throughout my nursing career who taught me so many lessons of life and of death. From my early days in medical-surgical nursing and pediatrics, to public health, oncology, clinical research, assisted living and hospice care, their stories have become the stories of my heart; those who died exactly the way they wanted and those who died in a way they neither planned for nor wanted. All of them live on in my mind and heart. I am honored to have known them and learned from them. It is my sincere hope that you who read this book make the vitally important decisions to ensure as much as possible your end of life care according to your wishes.

I am deeply grateful for the wisdom of many experts in the field of hospice and palliative care whose work inspired me as a nursing student in the 1970s and continues to shape the nurse and the person I am today. Dame Cicely Saunders and Elizabeth Kübler-Ross set me on my path toward palliative and hospice care with their passion to preserve the dignity of every individual at every stage of life from the moment of our birth to the moment of our death. Attending conference presentations by Dr. Byock and reading his engaging books further solidified my resolve to help people understand and plan for their own death. As a volunteer nurse at Capital Caring Hospice inpatient facility, Hank Dunn's gentle teachings energized me. Dr. Atul Gawande's book, Being Mortal, simply took my breath away. I read it and then reread it and am convinced it should be required reading for all of us who are going to die. The practical handbooks by Katy Butler and co-authors Dr. B.J. Miller and Shoshana Berger further galvanized my passion for a peaceful death revolution in our country. Drs. Paul and Lucy Kalanithe's life lessons they so eloquently and generously shared in the extraordinary book, When Breath Becomes Air, furthered my education in the experiences of death through physicians' eyes and hearts. I deeply admire Dr. Lucy Kalanithe's TedTalk on resilience following Paul's death and I keep her hard-won lessons close in my heart. Dr. Anthony Back taught me so much more than how to educate patients and families about the concept of prognosis when I was a content writer for the National Cancer Institute's cancer.gov website. His work as a medical communication educator and curriculum communications for the Center to Advance Palliative Care continues to inform and inspire me.

I owe huge thanks to my adult children and their families for their patience and encouragement of this book project. No doubt it is rather daunting to have a nurse mom and grandma focused as much on dying well as living well.

Finally, words fail me to fully express my infinite gratitude for my husband. His loving support, unfailing encouragement, and keen insights made this book possible.

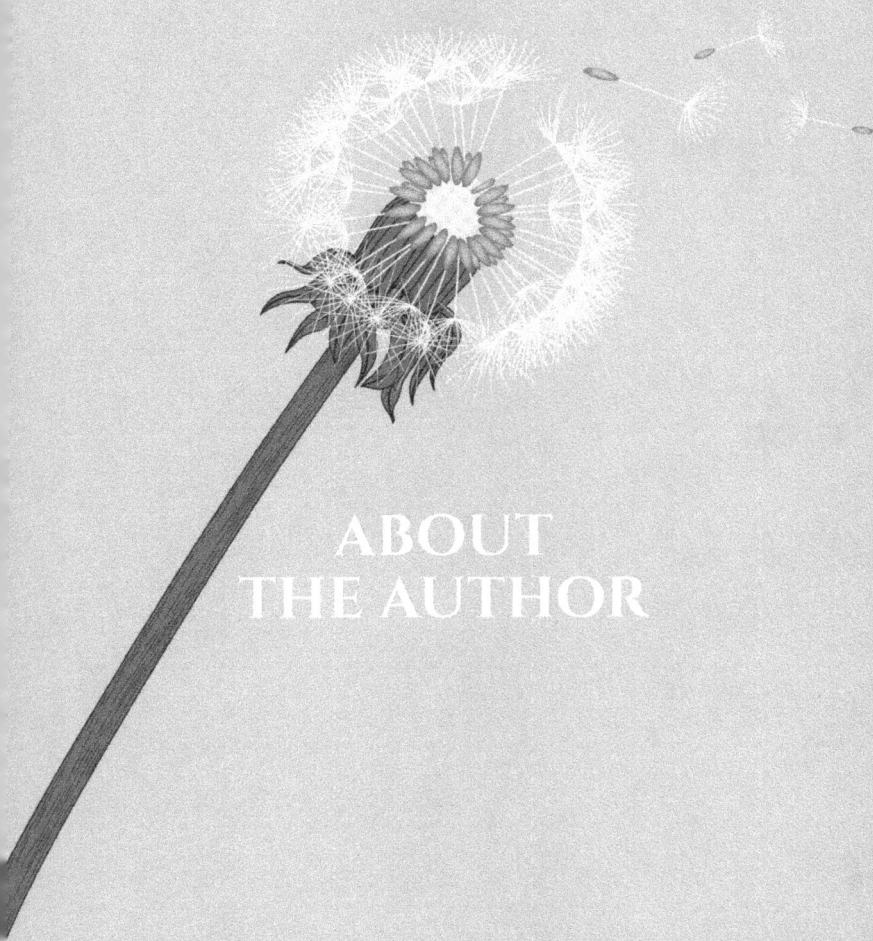

ABOUT
THE AUTHOR

ABOUT THE AUTHOR

Deborah (Deb) Price, RN, MSN, envisions a growing "peaceful death revolution" in which we all make our own fully informed choices as we contemplate and prepare for our inevitable death. She is a champion for choosing hospice care at end of life over acute care provided by hospitals.

Deb urges you to think about death before a health crisis makes you vulnerable to the "do everything" approach that often occurs in acute healthcare settings, the antithesis of the peaceful, comfortable death you may experience in your own home, surrounded by loved ones. Without proper planning, both the dying and their families risk heartbreaking guilt and regret instead of loving comfort at the end of life.

It is Deb's rally cry that we all can be more in control of our own lives until our last breath. Planning a good death is the ultimate last act of love for ourselves and for those we love.

Throughout her 45-year career in nursing (that included service in the USAF), Deb knew that providing quality care for the dying was the ultimate form of nursing for her. Inspired by Dr. Patch Adams and fellow nurse, Patty Wooten, Deb also became a therapeutic hospital clown (Nurse Hug-A-Bunch) to bring laughter to patients undergoing clinical research protocols. In addition to her work in clinical research, assisted living, and eldercare, Deb became certified in hospice and palliative nursing as well, and volunteered to provide care to patients in an inpatient hospice facility. She remains a member of the Hospice and Palliative Care Nurses Association. Her hospice experience and many other nursing experiences compelled her to write this book as a guide for everyone who is going to die.

Deb continues her work in health communication and science writing for the National Institutes of Health while she and her husband enjoy life in the foothills of the Blue Ridge Mountains in upstate South Carolina. For speaking inquiries, workshops, and just to connect, reach out to Deb at LovesLastAct@gmail.com.

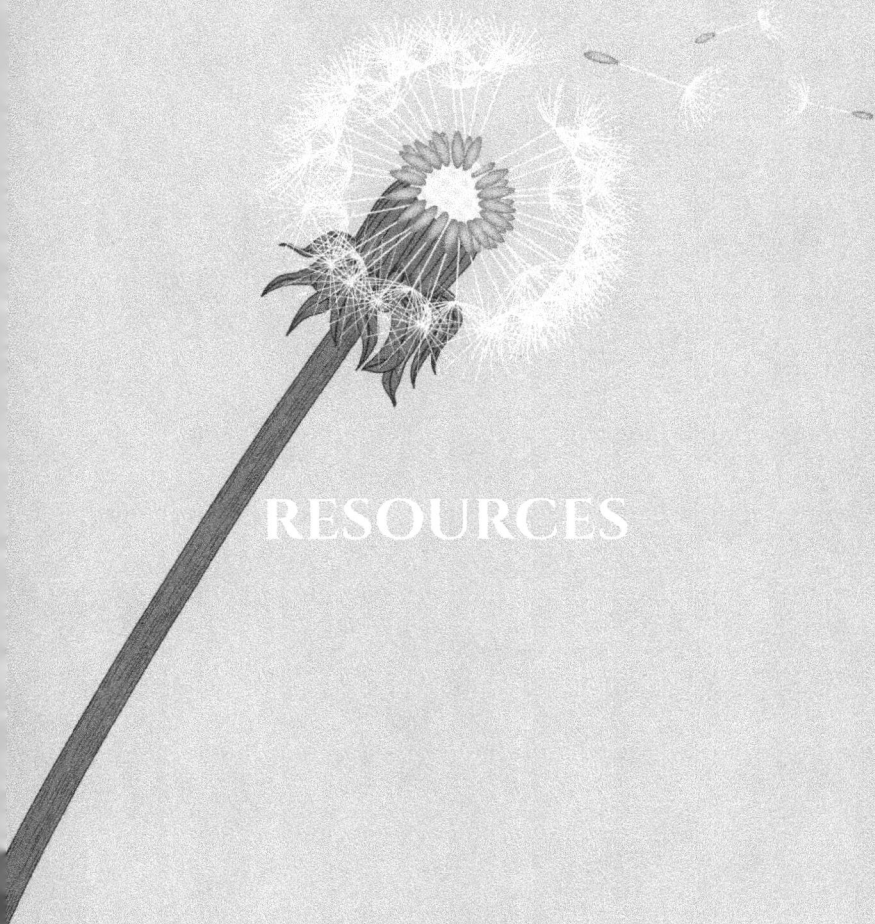

RESOURCES

RESOURCES

Advance Care Planning

Compassion and Choices
(compassion&choices.org)
Compassion & Choices is a U.S. nonprofit organization working to improve patient rights and individual choice at the end of life.
101 SW Madison Street, #8009
Portland, OR 97207
1-800-247-7421

Five Wishes—Advance Caring Planning Program
(fivewishes.org)
Five Wishes is a U.S. advance directive created by the nonprofit organization Aging with Dignity.
3050 Highland Oaks Terrace
Suite 2
Tallahassee FL 32301-3841
1-850-681-2010

National POLST Paradigm
(polst.org)
POLST is an approach to advance care planning for people who have a serious life-limiting medical condition or have advanced frailty and do not wish to have heroic measures if they suffer a medical crisis. The POLST form is a portable set of doctor's orders.
208 I Street NE
Washington, DC 20002
1-202-780-8352

Palliative Care

American Academy of Hospice and Palliative Medicine
(http://aahpm.org)
AAHPM is the professional organization for professionals specializing in hospice and palliative medicine.
1-847-375-4712

Palliative Doctors
(http://palliativedoctors.org)
PalliativeDoctors.org is the patient site of the American Academy of Hospice and Palliative Medicine (AAHPM). It is not intended to be a substitute for professional medical advice, diagnosis, or treatment but to provide as much information about hospice and palliative care as possible.

Center to Advance Palliative Care
(getpalliativecare.org)
CAPC is a national nonprofit organization dedicated to increasing the availability of quality health care for people facing serious illness. CAPC provides health care organizations with the tools, training, technical assistance and metrics needed to meet this need.
1-212-201-2670

Visiting Nurse Associations of America
(vnaa.org)
The VNAA is a nonprofit organization that supports, promotes, and advocates for the role of mission-driven home-based care providers including home health, hospice, and palliative care.
1-888-866-8773

Hospice

Hospice Foundation of America
(hospicefoundation.org)
HFA is nonprofit organization providing programs for professional development, public education and information related to advance care planning, hospice and palliative care, caregiving, and grief.
1701 L Street NW., Suite 220
Washington, DC 20036
1-202-457-5811

National Hospice and Palliative Care Organization
(nhpco.org)
NHPCO) is the largest U.S. nonprofit membership organization representing hospice and palliative care programs and professionals; committed to improving end-of-life care and expanding access to hospice care, and profoundly enhancing quality of life for people dying in America and their loved ones.
1731 King Street
Alexandria, VA 22314
1-800-658-8898 or 703-837-1500

Hospice Action Network
(hospiceactionnetwork.org)

CaringInfo
(nhpco.org)
CaringInfo, a program of the NHPCO that provides free resources to help people make decisions about end-of-life care and services before a crisis.

Services for Older Adults

AARP
(https://www.aarp.org)
AARP is a nonprofit, nonpartisan organization that empowers people to choose how they live as they age.
1-888-OUR-AARP
(1-888-687-2277)

Aging in Place
(https://www.aginginplace.org)
A resource for aging in place with information about achieving and maintaining optimal health, mobility, home modification, caregiving, finances, and technology.

National Directory of Home Modification and Repair Resources
(https://homemods.org)
The Fall Prevention Center of Excellence is a university-based, non-profit organization dedicated to promoting aging in place and independent living for persons of all ages and abilities; a resource for finding qualified local services and professionals to help modify and renovate your home for aging in place.

Eldercare Locator

(eldercare locator)

A public service of the U.S. Administration on Aging that offers care management services for older adults and their families.

1-800-677-1116

Elder Helpers

(elderhelpers.org)

National association of volunteers to help at home, provide transportation, help with shopping, cleaning, cooking, reading, writing, and simply keeping company.

My Healthfinder

(https://health.gov/myhealthfinder)

My Healthfinder is a service from the Department of Health and Human Services (HHS) that provides links to health-related websites, support, and self-help groups, plus links to government agencies and nonprofit organizations that assist seniors.

National Institute on Aging (NIA)

(https://www.nia.nih.gov)

NIA is dedicated to conducting research on aging as well as the health and well-being of older individuals. NIA offers topics for the elderly, information and news about the nature of aging and the aging process, and diseases and conditions associated with growing older.

Go4Life

(https://go4life.nia.nih.gov)

NIA's resource for exercise and physical activity designed to help you fit exercise and physical activity into your daily life.

Meals on Wheels America (MOW)

(https://www.mealsonwheelsamerica.org)
A meal program that operates in more than 5,000 independently-run local programs. Each community runs its Meals on Wheels based on the needs and resources of their communities to provide seniors with healthy meals in their own homes.
1-888-998-6325

Programs for All-Inclusive Care of the Elderly (PACE®)

(http://www.pace4you.org)
PACE assists people who are age 55 or older by providing and coordinating all the types of care for seniors living at home, including medical care, personal care, rehabilitation, social interaction, medications, and transportation. PACE seniors must be certified by their state to need nursing home care and live in a PACE service area (over 230 PACE centers in 31 states).
1-703-535-1565

Seniors Helping Seniors

(seniorshelpingseniors.com)
A national franchise company that matches seniors who need some help with other active seniors who want to provide help. Seniors who need help pay a reasonable hourly rate for whatever services they need. The seniors who help are paid a reasonable hourly wage for their service.

Senior Transportation Services

GoGo Grandparent
(gogograndparent.com)
Transportation services using Lyft or Uber for those without
a smartphone.

Veyo
(veyo.com)
Transportation service that partners with insurance companies
to provide seniors rides to medical appointments and for those
who need a special vehicle to accommodate a wheelchair
or stretcher. The service is free, providing the senior's health
insurance company includes Veyo as a transportation benefit.

ITN America
(itnamerica.org)
ITN America is a national non-profit senior transportation
network, from Maine to Florida to California.

Other Services

Assisted Senior Living
(https://www.assistedseniorliving.net)
One of the most comprehensive and unbiased directories
of senior care options searchable by state. Assisted Senior
Living was created by caregivers, for caregivers. Information
is from state and federal sources, combined with public
information to provide one of the most complete resources
for seniors and caregivers.

U.S. Department of Veterans Affairs—Veterans Health Administration

(https://www.va.gov/health/programs/index.asp)

A resource for military veterans including eligibility for benefits, optimizing health, compensated work therapy, disease prevention, prescriptions, caregiving, and living accommodation choices.

1-844-698-2311

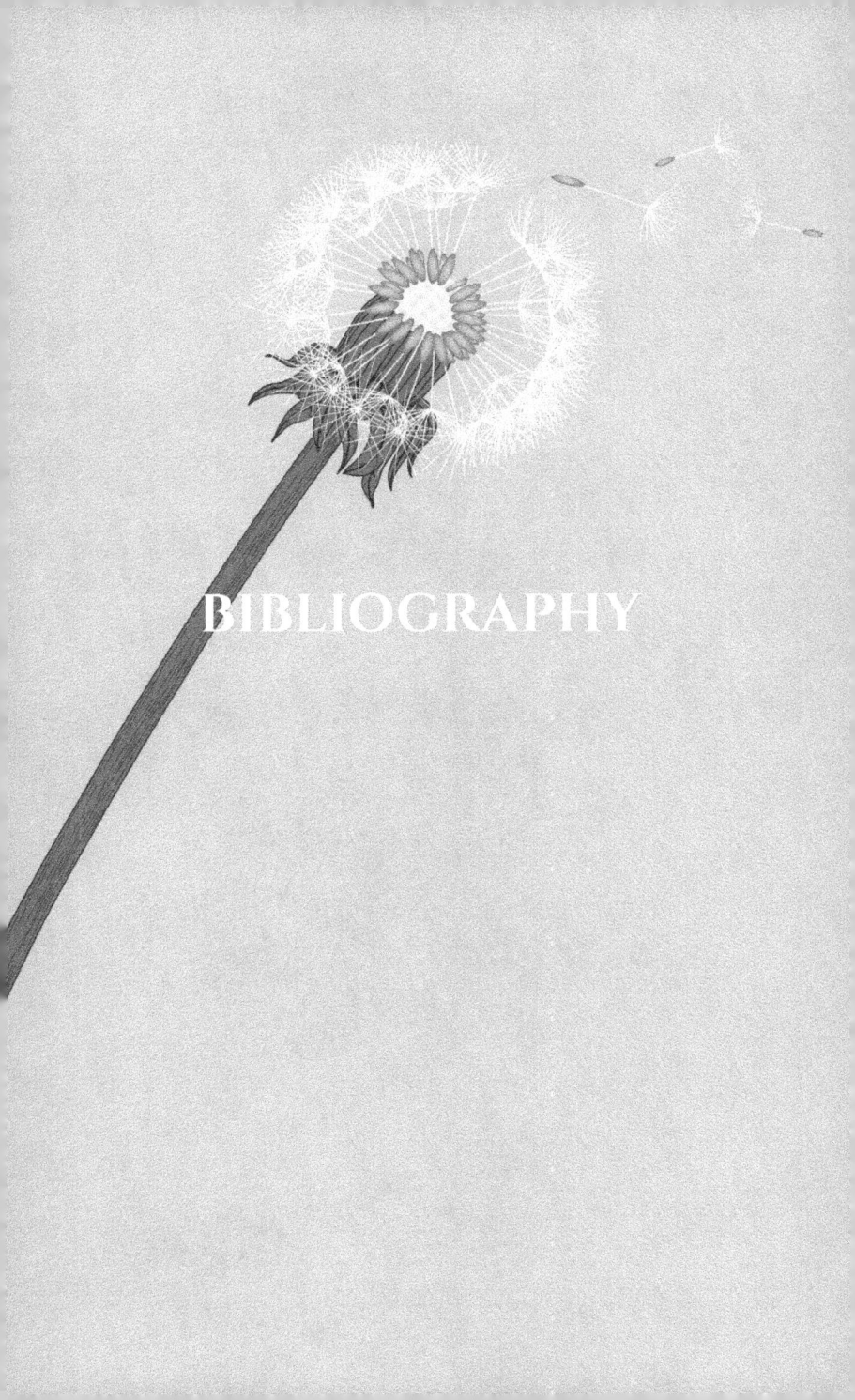

BIBLIOGRAPHY

BIBLIOGRAPHY

Byock, I., (1997). *Dying Well: Peace and Possibilities at the End of Life.* New York, NY: Riverhead Books-Penguin and Putnam.

Byock, I., (2014). *The Four Things That Matter Most: A Book About Living—10th Anniversary Edition.* New York, NY: Simon and Schuster.

Byock, I., (2014). *The Best Care Possible: A Physician's Quest to Transform Care Through the End of Life.* New York, NY: Penguin Group.

Byock, I., Kubler-Ross, E., (2014). *On Death and Dying: What the Dying Have to Teach Doctors, Nurses, Clergy, and their Own Families.* Fiftieth Anniversary Edition. New York, NY: Simon & Schuster/Scribner.

Buchwald. A., (2006) *Too Soon to Say Goodbye.* New York, NY: Random House.

Gawande, A., (2014). *Being Mortal: Medicine and What Matters in the End.* New York, NY: Metropolitan Books.

Dunn, H., (1990). *Hard Choices for Loving People.* Lansdowne, VA: A&A Publishers, Inc.

Kubler-Ross, E., (1969) *On Death & Dying*. New York, NY: Simon & Schuster/Touchstone.

NHPCO Facts and Figures (2018-Revision 7-2-2019). Alexandria, VA: National Hospice and Palliative Care Organization.

Banerjee, Rahul, MD., "Profanities, Promises, and Hospices." *Journal of Clinical Oncology* Volume 37. Issue 19 (2019): 1677-1679.

Miller, BJ., Berger, S., (2019) *A Beginner's Guide to the End: Practical Advice for Living Life and Facing Death*. New York, NY: Simon and Schuster.

Butler, K., (2019) *The Art of Dying Well: A Practical Guide to a Good End of Life*. New York, NY: Simon and Schuster.

Butler, K., (2014) *Knocking on Heaven's Door: The Path to a Better Way of Death*. New York, NY: Simon and Schuster.

Callahan, M. (2009) *Final Journeys: A Practical Guide to Bringing Care and Comfort to the End of Life*. New York, NY: Simon and Schuster.

Callahan, M., Kelley, P. (2012) *Final Gifts: Understanding the Special Awareness, Needs, and Communications of the Dying*. New York, NY: Simon and Schuster.

Kalanithe, P., (2016) *When Breath Becomes Air*. New York, NY: Random House.

National Center for Health Statistics, Kochanek KD, Murphy SL, Xu JQ, Arias E. Mortality in the United States, 2016. NCHS data brief, no 293. Hyattsville, MD: December 2017.

Creagan, E., MD (2018) Mayo Clinic on Healthy Aging. Rochester, MN, Mayo Clinic.

BIBLIOGRAPHY

Worden, J. William, (2018) *Grief Counseling and Grief Therapy: a handbook for the mental health practitioner.* New York, NY: Springer Publishing Company.

Neagle, Jayson T, MD, Wachsburg, Kelley, MD (2019) What Are the Chances a Hospitalized Patient will Survive In-Hospital Arrest?, *The Hospitalist.* 2010 September; 2010(9)